Side-Fx

Clinically relevant magic effects and tricks

for the health-care provider

D0354554

Side-Fx™

Clinically relevant magic effects and tricks
for the health-care provider

Scott Tokar and
Harrison J. Carroll

Side-Fx

Clinically relevant magic effects and tricks
for the health-care provider

By
Scott Tokar and Harrison J. Carroll

Published by Corporate-FX, Inc.
P.O. Box 1624 • Tustin, CA 92781
Printed in the United States of America

Edited by: Norma J. Collins, Tulsa, OK
Illustrations: Tony Dunn, Bonita Springs, FL
Cover Design: TheLooneyBin.com, Tustin, CA

Library of Congress Catalog Number 2004092065
ISBN 0-9749365-0-2

This publication is designed to provide accurate and authoritative
information with regard to the subject matter covered. It is sold
with the understanding that the publisher and authors are not en-
gaged in rendering medical, legal, accounting, or other professional
advice. If medical, legal advice or other expert assistance is required,
the services of a competent professional person should be sought.

From a *Declaration of Principles* jointly adopted by a committee
of the American Bar Association and a committee of Publishers
and Associations.

*This book is available at quantity discounts for bulk purchases.
For information, please call 1-800-624-4213*

DEDICATION

This endeavor is dedicated to the most wonderful
gift on our planet—CHILDREN.

And to two really precious gifts—Lucas and Stephanie.

CONTENTS

Scott Tokar, MIMC

S cott Tokar has been "playing" with magic tricks and kits since the early age of seven. As he grew, so did his love for magic. By the age of thirteen, he was performing regularly at children's birthday parties on weekends and after school. At the age of sixteen, Scott was accepted as a Junior Member in the elite group of magicians that form Hollywood's famous Magic Castle.

Under the guidance and supervision of some of magic's best-known names, Scott honed and perfected his craft. In 1988 Scott received the 1st place trophy for his intricate sleight of hand at the International Brotherhood of Magician's Conference held in Boston, Massachusetts.

After spending several years performing aboard cruise ships and in nightclubs, Scott began mixing his unique magic with a sales message. He then focused his career strictly on the corporate marketplace. In 1989 Scott assembled a team of corporate trade-show magicians called Corporate-FX. Today he can be found educating and enlightening audiences in trade shows, sales meetings, and conventions around the world.

Harrison J. Carroll, AIMC

At the age of eleven, Harrison and a boyhood friend pooled their allowances, hopped on a bus, and headed to the magic shop in downtown Buffalo, New York. There they bought a small trick and shared it, each one having it for a week before relinquishing it to the other. Little did Harrison know that these seeds of passion would eventually become his profession.

By the time he was eighteen, he was being schooled by some of the most distinguished sleight-of-hand artists of the day. In the mid-1970s he began performing magic professionally, and never looked back. He has worked with and performed for stars of film, television, literature, politics, athletics, and for people from every walk of life.

In 1982 he focused on offering his magical flair exclusively to the corporate culture. With a degree in marketing, it made perfect sense to combine magic with a company's desired message. Since that time he has performed at more than 500 trade shows and thousands of corporate events. His career has taken him to nearly every state and to thirteen countries.

. . . .

"Magic is—there's no other way to say it—magic...when it comes to instilling confidence and inspiration. Patients like to watch magic, and they love to learn to do it themselves. By imparting a skill even an "able-bodied" person doesn't have, you help patients acquire the assurance they need to persevere with a sense of determination and even joy. Magic's therapeutic benefits are not an illusion."

David Copperfield

. . . .

INTRODUCTION

Just about every parent has had the dreaded experience of dealing with a child's apprehension and anxiety during a visit to the doctor, dentist, or hospital facility.

In today's world of overloaded schedules and the hectic demands of high patient volume—with health-care professionals hastily grabbing charts and focusing on routine medical histories, ailments, or treatments—it can be easy to forget or just plain overlook a child's intimidation.

Think back for a moment to your own childhood visits to the doctor. Remember the overpowering sense of vulnerability that swept through your consciousness as you surveyed a roomful of odd-looking *things* that might be used to poke, prod, and hammer you? Do you remember gazing at that doctor in the odd-looking sci-fi coat, holding that giant needle that was about to stab you?

The practice of medicine has advanced by leaps and bounds through the years, but children's trepidations remain as real and intense as they were when your great grandparents were young. And, unfortunately, many of these conditioned fear responses can follow an individual all the way through adulthood and well into old age.

Traditionally, pediatricians have attempted everything they can—from hanging brightly colored posters on the wall to giving out lollipop rewards following successful exams—to alleviate the fears associated with a child's visit to the doctor. Today it's not unusual to find medical offices with elevated toy trains, Nickelodeon on the "big screen," and state-of-the-art video games in the waiting room. Anything that can be done to reduce patient stress can have a positive impact on a medical practice. Most likely, you have your favorite techniques already in place, and we don't want to change those. Our aim, through *Side-Fx*, is to provide you with new and unexpected methods that challenge you to think outside the box and ultimately make your patient interaction more productive, healing, and calming.

Many of the physicians involved in the creation of this book have told us that once they learned to invest a small amount of time in patient interaction up front, they realized immeasurable results in both productivity and satisfaction later on. By minimizing the unproductive time traditionally needed to calm a screaming, crying, or frightened child, these physicians were able to attend to their next patient sooner and in a more relaxed mood. In short, not only do they have happier patients, but their offices also become more efficient...and they tell us that they are able to end the day more joyfully and with less stress.

The purpose of this book is to provide you, the health-care professional, with tools and techniques specifically designed to divert a child's mind from the many fears associated with a visit to the doctor. By creating a surprise-filled, magical atmosphere for your patients, their habitual nervousness and concern are overcome by wonder and amazement.

We have spent countless hours researching, creating, and adapting a unique collection of illusions, puzzles, and conundrums specifically designed to assist health-care professionals in distracting and disarming apprehensive patients. In the following pages you will find numerous tricks, ploys, and gambits that are easy for you to perform and reproduce. The simple, magical methods outlined in the following pages should help put the little people you see in your practice at ease—and, hopefully, they'll see you more as a person and not as a terrifying mad scientist. Imagine transforming a troubled or even disorderly patient into a receptive, captivated, happy child who isn't undermining your goals but cheerfully facilitating them instead.

We are aware that the busy health-care provider doesn't have the time to collect props and learn intricate sleight-of-hand techniques. Therefore, we gathered effects that can be quickly mastered with everyday items found in most examining rooms and offices.

Although most of the effects are easy to do, and many require little or no practice, the material contained in this publication may not be applicable to each and every patient. Your personal judgment and experience will easily tell you which items will work best for particular ages and specific patient personalities. You may want to keep this book handy in your office for quick reference. But, rest assured, once you have learned and rehearsed an effect, you'll find that it will be easy to recall and successfully perform when that special situation arises.

We have attempted to simplify this book's layout to help you easily discover which mysteries will be the most clinically relevant for your practice at a particular moment in time. You'll find that our Icon Key will enable you to obtain a cursory overview of each effect's attributes. We have also included a simple rating system that will enable you to determine the degree of difficulty for each trick, as well as the amount of time needed to achieve its mastery. Each stunt has a brief "preface" to give you insight into how it may be relevant to your practice. The term "Fx" refers to "effect," which is, essentially, the effect as seen by the patient (observer). Many of the presentations feature a "professional tip" that adds deeper insight to the trick or its clinical application.

While writing *Side-Fx*, we originally envisioned a book focused solely on the pediatric patient. During development, however, physicians told us time and time again that many of these tricks are ideal relationship builders for use with all age groups and within a wide range of medical specialties. As an example, our trick *The Paralyzed Finger* is specifically targeted to help adult family members understand the frustration experienced by a cerebral palsy patient or a stroke victim. The effect *The Jumping Rubber Band* has a long history of being useful in connection with physical therapy through the Daniel Freeman Memorial Hospital program called "Project Magic." And radiological technicians just love the optical trick called *The Hole in the Hand,* which helps them explain the differences in diagnostic modalities available today.

With a little rehearsal and experience, we believe that you will start to create some awe and wonder in your own specialty. Relax, have fun, and allow yourself to be magical—and maybe your patients will actually look forward to the next time they get to visit their favorite "physician magician"!

ICON KEY

�֎ Rapport builder

➴ Familiarization with a medical device

⊕ Examination aid

🎲 Game

⧗ Time-saver

☑ You've just done the exam

✧ Clinical motor skill experiment

◗ Clinical reasoning and thinking assessment

☺ Just for fun

①-⑤ Skill level

    ① Easy; virtually no practice required.

    ② Requires minimal amount of practice.

    ③ Requires medium amount of practice.

    ④ Requires significant amount of practice.

    ⑤ Advanced; needs extensive preparation.

· ·

Warning: Throughout the book we recommend giving items used in various effects to the patient, as a souvenir or gift. Some of these objects are small and could be swallowed by small toddlers. When dealing with patients under the age of 3 years, we recommend NOT giving these items away—but, rather, making an effort to keep them out of the child's reach.

· ·

CHAPTER 1

The Waiting Patient

Time Killers for the Waiting Patient

A side from the anxiety created by waiting in an examining room, there can also be a substantial amount of boredom. Why not alleviate both by occupying the patient and/or guardian with some thought-provoking riddles and brainteasers?

The following items are surefire. Upon your entrance, you can check to see how the patient did—and if the puzzle was unresolved, you can quickly give the answer before proceeding with your exam.

The nurse or M.A. can use the paper from the examining table to write down these problems. Time spent waiting now passes much more quickly. This, according to the Direct Observation of Patient Care Case Study, increases your patient satisfaction.

You'll find more puzzles in the Swab Swami section on page 105.

Word Puzzles

✖   Rapport builder

⚀   Game

🗨   Clinical reasoning and thinking assessment

①   Skill level

. . . .

You will find the answers to these riddles on Page 205.

. . . .

1) Translate this: "YYURYYUBICURYY4ME."

2) Make this a sentence by adding only six pen strokes:

   "o o o o o o o o o o trick"

3) Make nine dots (three rows of three). Join all of the dots without lifting the pen and limiting yourself to only four strokes (moves) or less.

   0   0   0
   0   0   0
   0   0   0

4) What is this word?

   LEM
   AID

5) What is this?

   SIINFORMATIONDE

6) What is this?

   NNNNNNN
   AAAAAAA
   CCCCCCC

7) What is this?

   STAND
   I

CHAPTER 2

Unique Appearances

Entering the Examining Room

A n ideal way to make friends with the patient is to win them over right off the bat. A clever or unusual arrival can easily change the patient's chagrin or uncertainty into a huge smile.

Doorway Appearance

✖ Rapport builder

⧗ Time-saver

③ Skill level

PREFACE:

Sometimes there is an opportunity to build a friendly relationship with your patient even before you have entered the examining room. What do you do to break the ice when your patient is crying hysterically while waiting for you in the exam room? The answer is simple: Enter the room magically!

Fx:

As the exam room door swings open, the patient quickly notices that the caregiver is hanging from the doorjamb horizontally! The caregiver appears to possess super-hero-like powers as he or she remarkably climbs up and down the door frame at a 90° angle!

EXPLANATION:

You must try this effect to believe it! By assuming the posture represented in Diagram 1, your body really is at a 90° angle from the floor! But because your other foot (the one on the floor) is hidden from the view of the observer, the impression is that both of your feet are off the ground. It is important that you stick one of your legs *way* out to compensate for the one on the floor. Grab the doorjamb with both hands and "pull" yourself into view. You will look like a sideways "Kilroy Was Here" in real life. By bending your knee up and down, you can move your hands in a shuffle-like movement to make it look like you are literally climbing the walls to get in to see the next patient!

Diagram 1 shows the view from the patient's side of the wall. Diagram 2 exposes the method explained above.

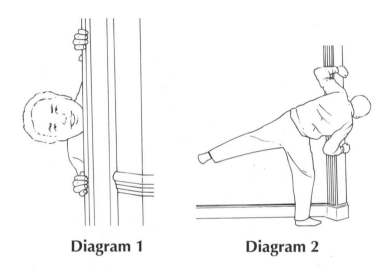

Diagram 1   **Diagram 2**

It will take a little practice to get the knack of it. But it is well worth the time invested and will prove to be an absolute winner with your pediatric patients.

PROFESSIONAL TIP:

The creator of this effect, Looy Simonoff, exudes a yell beforehand. The spectator sees one hand appear on the doorjamb, then the other hand. Finally, the head appears. The supporting leg is bent (putting his full weight on it). When he lets go with one hand and straightens the supporting leg, it creates the illusion of falling "upward," rather than across the wall. Finally, he falls "out" of the doorframe.

Doorway Puppet

✖   Rapport builder

✕   Time-saver

🎲   Game

①   Skill level

PREFACE:

If you've recently seen a movie at any chain movie theater, then you've seen the paper-bag puppets in the preshow advertisements. These are easy to make, and you are limited only by your own creativity and time.

FX:

A makeshift puppet can help you break the ice even before you enter the exam room. This is ideal for preschoolers. The hand puppet can ask the child patient what hurts, where it hurts, etc., thus making a game out of your evaluation while at the same time securing the information you need to help expedite your diagnosis.

EXPLANATION:

This is an ideal spur-of-the-moment solution to help calm the harried patient before you enter the room. By drawing a face on a paper lunch bag, as shown in Diagram 3, you can quickly fashion a puppet in no time!

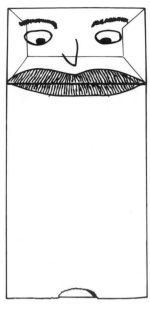

Diagram 3

You've just made a very portable hand puppet.

By opening and closing your hand, you can create the illusion of animation. The fictitious character can quickly befriend a child and even ask the necessary questions to aid in your diagnosis. *"What hurts?"* etc.

PROFESSIONAL TIP:

Preschoolers love to role-play and enter the world of make-believe. So don't underestimate the power of this simple tool. Some of the doctors we've talked to use an old sock instead of a paper bag. It makes less noise than the bag and lasts a lot longer.

CHAPTER 3

Items Likely to Be in the Examining Room

Cotton Ball Intrigue

In this section you will find effects accomplished with cotton balls. All the feats outlined rank high as rapport builders. They are designed to stimulate interaction with the child, while not consuming much time.

Guess Which Hand?

✖️ Rapport builder

💉 Familiarization with a medical device

🎲 Game

🗨️ Clinical reasoning and thinking assessment

① Skill level

PREFACE:

This is a fun way to determine a child's cognitive or deductive skills. Additionally, it is an excellent rapport builder, placing you in the position of being a fun person.

Fx:

The child fails to guess which hand secretly holds a cotton ball.

EXPLANATION:

Show a cotton ball in your right hand. Unknown to the child, you have a second cotton ball hidden in your left hand.

Place both hands behind your back as if to hide your actions from the child. Now bring both hands out in front of you and ask the child which hand the cotton ball is in. Whichever hand is indicated, open the other hand and say, *"Nope."*

Repeat the procedure until the child catches on. An analytical mind will quickly determine that you have a cotton ball in each hand. The last thing you want is for the patient to feel foolish. Rather, you want to leave them with a sense of accomplishment. Let the child catch you. Attitude is the key to success!

PROFESSIONAL TIP:

Once the child has deduced that you have two cotton balls, his or her self-esteem is elevated. This puts you in a better position to interact directly with the patient, and not solely the accompanying guardian.

. . . .

"It's amazing how easy these items are to learn, and how quickly they allow you to break the ice with the apprehensive child. I wish this book was required reading at medical school years ago."

Hector Ramirez, M.D.
Rancho Santa Margarita, CA

. . . .

Jumping Cotton Balls

♛ Rapport builder

🔪 Familiarization with a medical device

② Skill level

PREFACE:

As indicated above, this effect will require a little practice. But it is well worth the fifteen minutes or so needed to become comfortable hiding the extra object in your hand. It is superior to the previous piece in that its method is more inexplicable.

Fx:

A cotton ball impossibly passes from your pocket and appears inside the patient's clenched hand.

EXPLANATION:

For this piece you will need four cotton balls. Place them in the right pocket of your lab coat or pants.

When you are ready to perform, reach into the pocket with your right hand and secure all four balls. Remove your hand, bringing it in front of you. Now the left hand reaches into the right and extracts three balls, leaving one behind. The ball not taken remains unknown to the patient. It stays concealed in the right hand, hidden from view because the back of the hand is always toward the patient. Diagram 4 shows the three cotton balls in the left hand and exposes the hidden ball in the right.

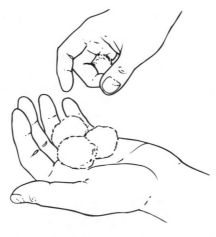

Diagram 4

Note: If you keep your fingers curled up slightly, the patient won't suspect that you have a cotton ball inside it. But you will want to keep all attention on the *left* hand as you ask the spectator to place his or her right hand out, palm up, as shown in Diagram 5.

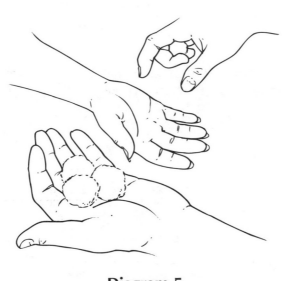

Diagram 5

Now your right hand (still concealing the ball) picks up one of the cotton balls from your left hand and deposits it into the palm of the spectator's hand, as illustrated in Diagram 6.

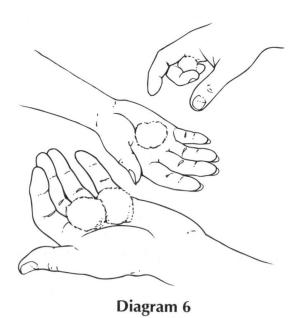

Diagram 6

Ask your spectator assistant what is in his or her left hand. The child will say, "A cotton ball." Then ask, *"How many did you say?"*

The patient will reply, "One."

Now, with the right hand, remove the ball from the child's hand and ask again, *"How many do you have now?"*

The reply will be, "None."

Say, *"I'll give it back, but hold it real tightly."*

As you say this, redeposit the cotton ball just removed, but also add the hidden cotton ball. Once the balls are added, immediately use your empty right hand to assist in closing the spectator's hand tightly. You must forcibly aide the patient in closing his or her hand. Otherwise, the child could prematurely open it and see the added cotton ball.

The spectator now has two cotton balls, but thinks there is only one. Affirm this by saying, *"You have one cotton ball, and I have two."*

Continue by openly putting one of your two cotton balls back into your pocket. Say, *"If I place one in my pocket, I can magically cause it to fly into your hand. Watch!"*

Suiting the action to the words, place the ball into your pocket, then bring your empty hand out and make a magic pass.

Have the child open his or her hand to find the two cotton balls. After it has sunk in, grab all the remaining cotton balls and place them in your pocket or a nearby trash can.

One through Ten

�֎ Rapport builder

⚲ Familiarization with a medical device

🗨 Clinical reasoning and thinking assessment

⧗ Time-Saver

② Skill level

PREFACE:

A little practice will go a long way in making this one a winner for you. It happens very quickly (as long as it takes you to count to ten). This is a very fast method of taking the child's mind away from the confusing surroundings and making him more amenable to your upcoming exam.

Fx:

After a series of hand maneuvers, a cotton ball seems to magically pass from one hand to the other.

EXPLANATION:

The key to success is in the cadence and rhythm of the counting sequence. There is a crucial *move* that you will need to become comfortable with. But you should easily master it in less than fifteen minutes.

Place two cotton balls on the examining table, about six inches apart, next to the patient. See Diagram 7.

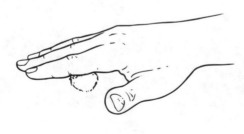

Diagram 7

Ask the patient to watch, and begin your patter (counting to ten) in a rapid, smooth pattern from one to ten. As each number is recited, a specific action must be taken.

"One." Rest your open right hand, palm down, on top of the cotton ball that is to your right. Your palm should lightly contact the cotton ball, as shown in Diagram 8.

Diagram 8

"Two." Rest your open left hand, palm down, on top of the cotton ball that is to your left. Your palm should also lightly contact the cotton ball. See Diagram 9.

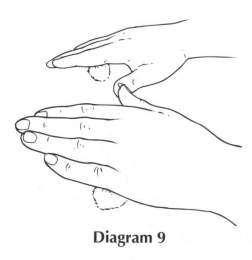

Diagram 9

"Three." Turn your right hand over. Now the back of the hand gently contacts the ball. Your position should replicate that shown in Diagram 10.

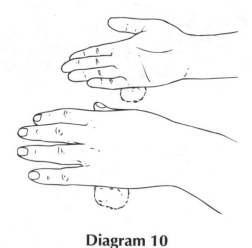

Diagram 10

"Four." Turn your left hand over. Now the back of this hand gently contacts the ball. See Diagram 11.

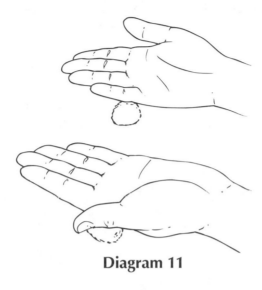

Diagram 11

"Five." Lift your right hand. Turn it over and pick up the cotton ball, lifting it about three inches off the table, with the right fingertips and thumb. Keep the left hand where it is. See Diagram 12.

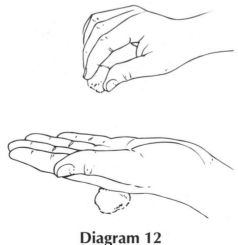

Diagram 12

"Six." Now the crucial *move* mentioned earlier. Move your right hand to the left hand (still palm up). You will pretend to place the cotton ball, held in the right hand, into the left hand, but you don't. Instead, three things happen.

First, the right hand comes to the left hand, stopping when the cotton ball contacts the left palm. Second, the right-hand thumb slides the cotton ball from the fingertips down into the fingers. Your position should resemble the illustration in Diagram 13.

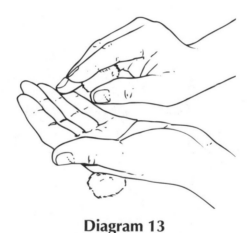

Diagram 13

Finally, the left hand closes as if it were clenching the deposited cotton ball. See Diagram 14.

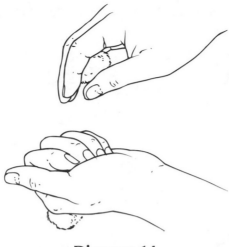

Diagram 14

Without interrupting your cadence, continue. *"Seven."* The left hand moves further to the left, fully revealing the ball that was beneath it. The right-hand fingers simultaneously snatch the cotton ball from the table (previously under the left hand). See Diagram 15. The right fingers then close around the cotton balls.

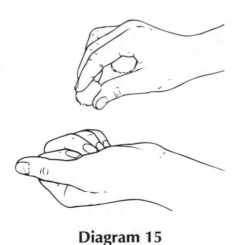

Diagram 15

"Eight." Turn both hands up so the backs of the palms rest on the table, as shown in Diagram 16.

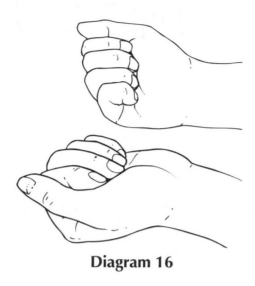

Diagram 16

"Nine." Open the left hand and show that it is empty, as shown in Diagram 17.

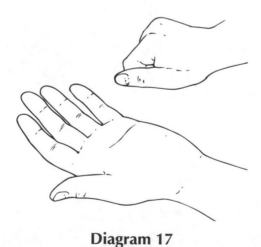

Diagram 17

"Ten." Turn the right hand over and open it to reveal both cotton balls, as shown in Diagram 18.

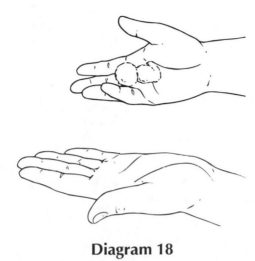

Diagram 18

Let them drop to the table. It's all as easy as counting One to Ten.

PROFESSIONAL TIP:

We went to great lengths to describe what takes ten seconds to perform. That's because we believe that this is a "gem" that will captivate the child patient. The really young children will count along with you because they love to show off their counting skills. As they count, they'll watch in amazement when the cotton ball ends up in the other hand.

When you first practice, it is natural that your counting sequence will "hang up" at six. But after a few run-throughs you'll start getting the hang of it. Ideally, you do NOT want to break the counting rhythm at six. You want to achieve a smooth, rapid, count. Before you know it, it will be as easy as, well... counting to ten!

Small children love to show off their ability to count to ten. We advise you to encourage them to count along with you. It serves two purposes:

1) It provides a perfect way to align yourself with the patient, in order to make him or her more amenable to your upcoming exam.

2) It focuses the child's mind on the counting procedure rather than trying to figure out what you're up to.

. . . .

"You will not only leave your patients happy and mesmerized. But, it's more likely they will get better because they will be prone to follow the suggestions of their magic doctor."

Randolph Cordle, M.D., F.A.C.E.P., F.A.A.P., P.E.M.
Pediatric and Adult Emergency Medicine
Carlisle, PA

. . . .

Wolves and Sheep

✖   Rapport builder

➤   Familiarization with a medical device

◀   Clinical reasoning and thinking assessment

①   Skill level

PREVIEW:

Not only will this amaze your patient, but also it comes with a great little story that is guaranteed to relax the patient and get his or her mind off the thought of visiting the doctor.

Fx:

The effect of this piece is best explained as the story progresses. So follow along.

EXPLANATION:

Begin by laying seven cotton balls in a row, on the examining table next to the patient. Pick up one cotton ball in each hand and display them with your palms up and open.

Say, *"There once were two wolves."*

Show the cotton ball in your left hand and say, *"This is Binky."* Show the cotton ball in your right hand and say, *"This is Winky."* See Diagram 19.

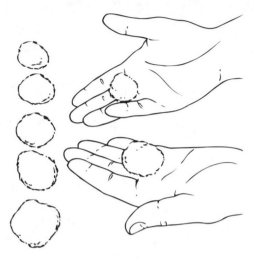

Diagram 19

Continue: *"They were hiding behind a hill when they saw five sheep. Binky said to Winky, 'Let's get those sheep.'"*

Close your hands into fists, hiding the "wolves" from view. Pick up one of the sheep (cotton balls) with your left hand and pick up one with your right hand. Continue picking up the cotton balls until you have all five. The last cotton ball should be picked up by your left hand, giving you more cotton balls in that hand than in the right.

On with the story: *"Binky said to Winky, 'Did you hear somebody coming? I think it's the sheepdog. We better put these sheep back until he is gone.'"*

Without opening your hands, drop one cotton ball from your right hand onto the table. Simultaneously, do the same with the left hand. Continue doing this until there are five cotton balls back on the table.

Your right hand should be empty, but keep both hands closed as if they both held cotton balls. Say, *"So those wolves waited, and when they were sure there was no sheepdog coming..."*

Shake your right fist and say, *"Winky said, 'Binky,'* (shake your left fist) *'you dummy. There was no sheepdog. Let's steal those sheep and go home.'"*

Starting with your left hand, pick up the cotton balls as before—alternating hands throughout the pick-up. Upon completion, your right hand should have two cotton balls, and your left hand should have five.

Complete your story. *"So they picked up the sheep and went home. But there was a problem. The sheepdog really was there, after all. He followed those wolves all the way home. And that sheepdog stole those sheep right back from those wolves and took them back to the field."*

Open your right hand and show two pieces of cotton. *"Winky and Binky were all alone. What about the sheep?"* Open your left hand and show the five pieces of cotton.

PROFESSIONAL TIP:

The story will be as amusing as the visual discovery. More importantly, it provides the physician with an ideal way to introduce cotton balls that might be used for any number of purposes.

Tongue Blade Enigmas

The tongue blade can be used for a variety of entertaining and intriguing experiences, all guaranteed to generate a huge smile on the patient's face. As with the cotton balls from the previous section, you are familiarizing the patient with a medical device. This makes it less foreign and less threatening to them.

Making Smiles

✖ Rapport builder

➤ Familiarization with a medical device

ⓧ Examination aid

② Skill level

PREFACE:

When Scott first started practicing magic at the age of seven, the *paddle move* was one of the first *sleights* in his repertoire. It is a simple move, and can be learned by anyone in a matter of minutes.

Fx:

A tongue blade (tongue depressor) is shown to be blank on both sides, but with a flick of the wrist a smiley face magically appears on both the front and the back!

EXPLANATION:

When doing the *paddle move*, you pretend to show both sides of the tongue blade, but in reality you are just showing the same side twice. An optical illusion principle called *visual assumption* causes the brain to accept that the tongue blade is normal, or blank, on both sides.

First, it may be helpful to actually try the un-magical movement that is being mimicked in this trick. Mark one side of a tongue blade with a happy face. In a mirror, practice displaying both sides of the tongue blade by simply turning your wrist with a radial motion. The wrist should not move from left to right, but simply rotate. First display one side, and then show the other side by rotating your wrist only 180°. As you do this, one side will show as blank and the other will show the happy face. See Diagrams 20 and 21, illustrated with the tongue blade in the left hand.

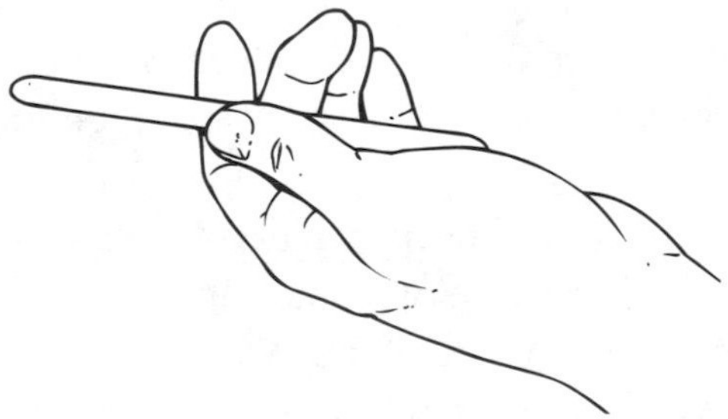

Diagram 20

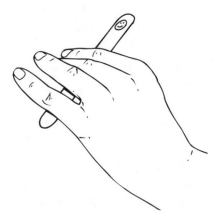

Diagram 21

Next, try the magical *move*. For this effect you must learn to "flip" the tongue blade at the tips of your fingers. By holding the tongue blade at the tip of your middle fingers and thumb, as outlined in Diagram 20, it is easy to simply "flip" it over with your thumb while simultaneously turning your wrist. The object is to make the move look (as closely as possible) just like the un-magical move we discussed at the beginning.

The fact that the thumb is flipping the tongue blade in order to show the same side twice will pass unnoticed by the larger movement of the tongue blade itself. Practice this move a few times so that you can get familiar with the action and the feeling of this "flip." Again, all you are attempting to do here is to turn the tongue blade 180° at the tips of your fingers to show the same side, but you are giving the appearance of showing both sides. Upon completing the action, your hand should resemble the position shown in Diagram 22.

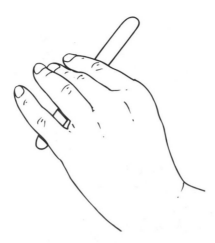

Diagram 22

Once the maneuver is complete, you will have created an impression of showing both sides. It is very disarming.

Practice this move in front of a mirror a few times, and soon you will be convincing yourself that the tongue blade is blank on both sides. To make the smiley face ☺ magically appear, simply use the radial wrist movement *without* adding the thumb/index finger "flip move." Once again, repeat the flip rotation to show the patient that the smiley face has appeared on both sides!

Patter:

Display the tongue blade as blank on both sides, and say, *"Hello Timmy. I understand that you have a bit of a sore throat today—is that true? Well, if you will let me have a quick look, I'll bet I can make you a happy face."* Turn the tongue blade to make the smiley face magically appear.

PROFESSIONAL TIP:

The *paddle move*, once mastered, is fun to do and actually feels good to perform. However, don't "over prove" it by showing each side over and over. In performance, you should display one side of the tongue blade only once or twice. If you are standing there in front of a patient and turning an apparently blank tongue blade over and over in your hands, the patient is liable to look more closely at your actions and eventually catch that there is some kind of tricky motion going on. Given enough opportunity to study your movements, any spectator will catch you red-handed (and red-faced)! Try this: *"Look! The stick is blank on this side and on this side. See? But by saying a magical word, 'Acute Bacterial Otitis Media'* (do the flip move), *you'll see that Mr. Smiley face appears right on the stick."* Then put the tongue blade away. Or you may wish to give it to the patient as a souvenir. In either case, you're ready to retrieve a fresh tongue blade and continue with your exam.

Also, watch your viewing angles and note the pivot point of the tongue blade at your fingertips. Practice this move in a mirror to see for yourself what it will look like to the patient; some angles look better than others.

The Name Game

✖ Rapport builder

➤ Familiarization with a medical device

⊕ Examination aid

② Skill level

Fx:

A tongue blade is shown to be blank on both sides. But upon closer inspection, the child's name magically appears on one side. The tongue blade is definitely given to the child as a souvenir from the magical doc! As with the last effect, grab a fresh tongue blade for your exam.

EXPLANATION:

This effect uses the exact same movements that you just learned in the previous ploy, the *paddle move*. However, instead of using a smiley face, you simply write the child's name on one side before you enter the exam room. Just obtain the name from the child's chart, write the name on one side of the tongue blade, and you are ready to perform. Don't write small. Fill a large area of the tongue blade, as shown in Diagram 23.

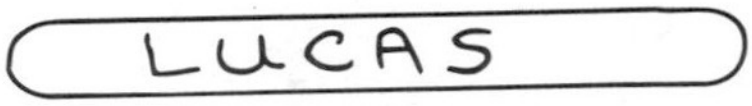

$$\boxed{\text{L U C A S}}$$

Diagram 23

PROFESSIONAL TIP:

In both cases, if age appropriate, let the child keep the tongue blade as a souvenir.

. . . .

"Giving out toys and performing magic makes the visit to the physician special. For many children it helps to relieve the anxiety of a visit to the doctor. And, isn't it our job as physicians and pediatricians to treat the patient and not just the disease?"

Gilbert I. Furman, M.D.
Covina, CA

. . . .

Magnetized Stick

✘   Rapport builder

✒   Familiarization with a medical device

⊕   Examination aid

①   Skill level

PREVIEW:

This is a quick stunt that will assuredly grab the patient's attention. It's another great way to introduce the tongue blade, and it provides a perfect transition to your oral examination.

FX:

A tongue blade seems to remain suspended against the palm of your hand.

EXPLANATION:

A picture is worth a thousand words. Diagrams 24 and 25 fully explain the ruse behind the illusion.

Let the spectator see you close your left fingers around the tongue blade. Then turn the back of your hand toward the patient. With the right hand, grab hold of your left wrist. In doing so, allow your right index finger to run parallel to your left forearm. Now slide your right hand upward and push your right index finger into the closed left hand until it contacts the tongue blade. Press the tip of the right finger against the tongue blade, securing it in place. Now open your fingers. The position shown in Diagram 24 is an exposed view.

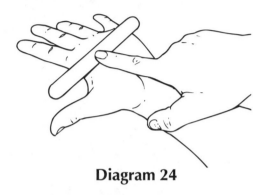

Diagram 24

What the spectator sees is illustrated in Diagram 25.

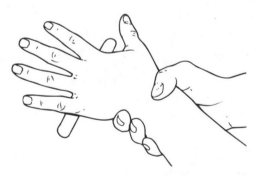

Diagram 25

PROFESSIONAL TIP:

Once the illusion is set in the patients mind, instruct the child to hold out his or her hands—release the pressure applied to the tongue blade by your right index finger and allow gravity to let it drop into the patient's waiting palms.

We've been told by many doctors that this is an excellent item to teach the child's parent. And don't forget—give the child the tongue blade as a memento, if age appropriate.

. . . .

"It makes great sense to use these simple techniques to create a friendly atmosphere in the office or hospital. I use items such as this to calm nervous kids, which greatly speeds up my examination time."

Robert W. Block, M.D.
Professor and Daniel C. Plunket Chair
Department of Pediatrics, University of Oklahoma, Tulsa, OK

. . . .

Three Choices

- Familiarization with a medical device
- Examination aid
- ① Skill level

PREVIEW:

This effect requires a little advance preparation. But once done, you will be set for a long time. We've listed it under tongue blades, even though you'll need two other items.

First: With a magic marker, write the following on the back side of a tissue box:

"You Will Choose This Box."

Second: Write the following on the back side of a box of exam gloves:

"You Will NOT Choose This Box."

Finally: Write the following on the back side of a canister or a box of tongue blades:

"You Will NOT Choose This Box."

See Diagrams 26, 27, and 28.

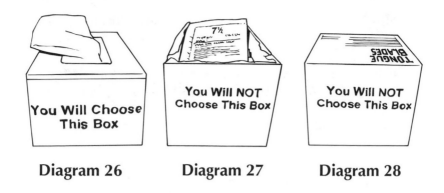

| Diagram 26 | Diagram 27 | Diagram 28 |

It's that easy, and you are set to perform. Once you become fluent with your presentation, you can change the chosen item to set you up for your next exam. We'll talk about this later. For now, let's look at the effect.

Fx:

The three items are placed on the examining table, next to the seated patient. The patient ends up with the box of tissue every time.

EXPLANATION:

With the items placed next to the patient, ask the child to pick up two items. What you say next will depend on which items are picked up. And you will have to be ready to give different instructions accordingly. (So you will have to do a little mental practice on this one. But it is very easy, and you should have it down in no time.)

All possible scenarios are covered here:

1) If the patient picks up the box of tongue blades and the gloves, immediately say, *"And hand them to me."* There should be virtually no pause between your instruction

---

to pick them up and your second instruction to hand them to you.

2) If the patient picks up the tissue box and either of the other items, immediately say, *"And hand one to me."*

Now he or she can hand you either the tissue box or the other item.

First: If the patient hands you the tissue box, say, *"Okay, and you can set the other box to the side."* Then explain that out of all three items, he or she gave you the correct one. Turn the box around and show the writing. Don't worry about showing the writing on the other items. The patient will probably check that out.

Second: The patient will hand you a wrong item, keeping the tissue box. Say, *"Are you sure?"* When the answer is, "Yes," place the other item aside and ask him or her to read the back side of the tissue box. Again, don't worry about showing the back sides of the other items. Either your patient will do it or ask you to show it.

PROFESSIONAL TIP:

The key to success in this piece is to convey each option in a steady cadence. Your delivery should be smooth and precise. After a few tries, you'll have it mastered.

Once you are comfortable with your presentation, you can expand your horizons. It becomes a simple matter to change the *forced* item to be anything you wish. You may make the tongue blades box the item of choice, providing a perfect segue to removing one and asking the child to *"Open wide."*

Make sure the writing is away from the view of the patient.

Termites

- Familiarization with a medical device
- Examination aid
- Just for fun
- ① Skill level

PREVIEW:

This is a quickie that provides a nice transition to examining the patient's throat.

FX:

You explain that there are termites in your wooden stick (tongue blade). The child patient hears them running through the wood.

EXPLANATION:

Hold the tongue blade to the patient's ear but away from his or her vision. Now simply scratch the surface of the tongue blade with your fingernail. See Diagram 29. The patient will hear the termites.

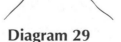

Diagram 29

Paper Cup Magic

If you don't have a paper cup dispenser in your office or examining room, this one may not be for you. However, after reading these effects you may want to install one.

Floating Paper Cup

- ⚒ Rapport builder
- ⧗ Time-saver
- ☺ Just for fun
- ① Skill level

PREVIEW:

This requires a little advance preparation, but it is very minor and easy to do. Simply make two cuts in the cup to form an X. Make each cut slightly less than an inch long. See Diagram 30. Now place the cup back into the dispenser.

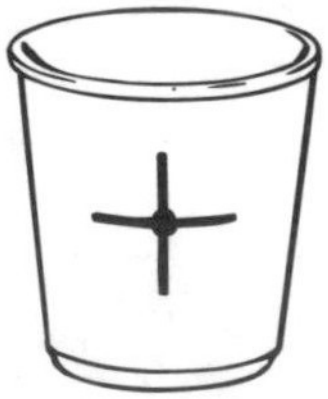

Diagram 30

Fx:

When the moment is right, show the patient your ability to make things float. Remove your prepared cup from the dispenser. Hold it casually, with the precut side of the cup facing your chest.

Standing in front of the patient, re-grip the cup by the sides. Secretly insert your left thumb into the carved-out X. Once secure, move your hands apart, as shown in Diagram 31. The cup appears to be floating in midair between your hands.

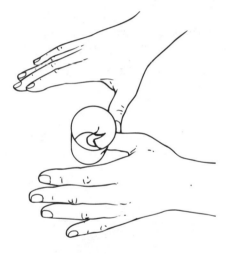

Diagram 31

Make sure to point your thumb directly at the patient's line of sight. The view from the patient's perspective is outlined in Diagram 32.

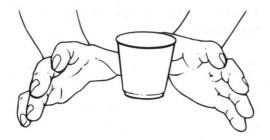

Diagram 32

After a few seconds, grab the cup with both hands and pull it back. You may want to comment about its floating ability as you crumple the cup and toss it in the trash can.

PROFESSIONAL TIP:

This trick is a natural for dentists. Before asking the patient to rinse, make the cup float.

Topsy-Turvy Cups

✖ Rapport builder

⚅ Game

🗩 Clinical reasoning and thinking assessment

① Skill level

PREVIEW:

This is a thought-provoking puzzle that is ideal for those inquisitive preteen patients.

FX:

As we mentioned, this is a puzzle. It is designed to challenge the patient's problem-solving ability, and it can be used to occupy his or her time while you are out of the room.

EXPLANATION:

Assume the child is seated on the examining table for a follow-up visit for some minor ailment.

Remove three cups from your paper cup dispenser and set them next to the patient on the examining table, in the following manner: The two cups on the ends are mouth-down and the middle one is mouth-up. See Diagram 33. The cups are labeled A, B, and C for easy reference.

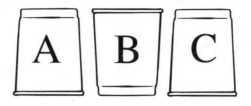

Diagram 33

Instruct the patient on the following rules:

Rule #1: After three turns, all the cups must be mouth-up.

Rule #2: Cups must be turned over two at a time.

Rule #3: Each cup must be turned over at least one time.

Rule #4: Three turns, and only three turns, must be used to solve the problem.

Demonstrate how <u>not</u> to perform by turning A and C without turning B. Explain that this solution is not correct because cup B hasn't been turned.

Remember: two cups at a time must be turned over so that if those cups were upside down, they will now be right side up (or vice versa—if they were right side up, they would now be upside down). Three of these double turns must be made, and upon the conclusion, all the cups must be mouth-up. After the patient fails to successfully attain the final position of having all three cups mouth-up, show him or her how easy it is.

The secret to a triumphant conclusion is shown in Diagram 36. For the first move, turn over cups A and B. Once completed, the positions should be as shown in Diagram 34.

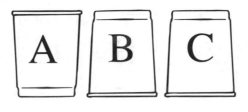

Diagram 34

For the second move, turn over cups A and C. That will leave the positions as shown in Diagram 35.

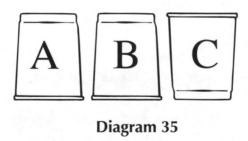

Diagram 35

For the third move, simply repeat your initial actions, turning over cups A and B. If everything was done correctly, your arrangement should be the same as the cups shown in Diagram 36.

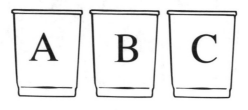

Diagram 36

PROFESSIONAL TIP:

Obviously, this is not for the preschooler but is recommended for the older child.

. . . .

**Remember to visit
http://www.SideFxMagic.com**

. . . .

How Deep Is My Cup?

✖ Rapport builder

😊 Just for fun

🔊 Clinical reasoning and thinking assessment

① Skill level

PREVIEW:

This stunt requires a tongue blade and a paper cup. That's all you need, and you'll be amazing the patient in no time.

FX:

You prove that the inside of the paper cup (or any cup) is deeper than the outside.

EXPLANATION:

Hold the cup in the left hand and place the tongue blade in your right, as illustrated in Diagram 37. Note the position of the right thumb.

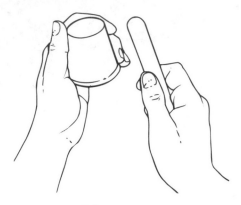

Diagram 37

Tell the patient that you will measure the inside of the cup by using the stick. Insert the tongue blade into the cup, and use your right thumb to mark the edge of the cup, as shown in Diagram 38.

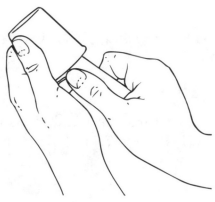

Diagram 38

When you remove the tongue blade, let your right arm lower. As you do, slide your thumb about an inch down the tongue blade, as shown in Diagram 39. The child will not notice this subtle maneuver.

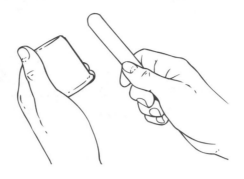

Diagram 39
Notice that the thumb slides down

Now hold the tongue blade adjacent to the exterior of the cup, as shown in Diagram 40, bringing your thumb to the bottom edge. The tongue blade will extend over the top of the cup, proving that the inside is deeper than the outside.

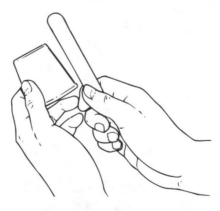

Diagram 40

PROFESSIONAL TIP:

Although this may seem silly, the child will be confounded, and it's a good lead-in to any exam or medical procedure that involves a tongue blade. It is quick and easy to accomplish. One doctor told us that she uses this trick before asking for a urine sample, reminding her patients not to spill it.

Otoscopes and Specula

That familiar speculum is about to offer you a perfect entrée to an ENT exam. The odd-looking otoscope and speculum can easily be used to create some magic, easing the child's trepidations before an ear exam.

The 45-Second ENT Exam

✘   Rapport builder

✎   Familiarization with a medical device

☑   You've just done the exam

✪   Examination aid

⌛   Time-saver

③   Skill level

PREVIEW:

This piece uses an old magician's sleight-of-hand move known as a *Thimble Vanish*. A variation of the old *Quarter-in-the-Ear* trick, this illusion specifically uses a speculum from an otoscope. By repeating the effect twice, the doctor turns an otherwise purely clinical exam into a fun, magical game. More importantly, the exam is being conducted at the same time. In many cases, this approach to the ENT exam can turn an otherwise screaming, uncooperative child into a giggling, obliging one in fewer than 45 seconds!

This will require a little practice on your part, but you'll find it well worth the investment.

Fx:

The physician introduces a speculum, places it onto the tip of his finger, and causes it to vanish. The speculum is found, with a magical flair, inside the patient's ear. The trick is repeated once again—only this time, even though the doctor expects to find it in the same ear, it seems to have vanished to some other place. To locate the speculum and illuminate the ear, the doctor uses his magic light (an otoscope), first to look in one ear and then the other…and then to look in the nose and mouth. Suddenly it dawns on the doctor that it was on the end of his light (the otoscope) the entire time! The mischievous speculum (thimble) can then be given to the child as a magical souvenir.

It is important for us to mention the obvious. *A chocking hazard exists when small children play with small parts and toys. We advise keeping track of the speculum and making sure it is not given to children under three years of age.*

EXPLANATION:

The first step is to prepare all the otoscopes in your examining rooms. Simply place a speculum onto each otoscope. Place it back in its holder, and you're set to go.

The *Thimble Vanish* is relatively easy to perform once you are familiar with the physical motions and the feel of the speculum in your hands.

First, place the speculum on your right index finger. Make a loose fist with your left hand. Put the speculum and your index finger into the closed fist, as shown in Diagram 41.

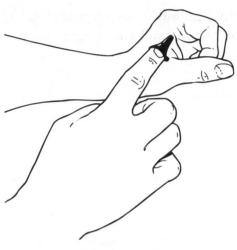

Diagram 41

At this point you *could* tighten the grip of your left hand. The spectator will believe that you left the speculum in your closed left fist. However, you are not going to tighten your fist. To the contrary, you are going to make a very loose fist, allowing you to curve your index finger (and the speculum) back around the left thumb. Diagram 42 reflects this action from behind, with the right thumb moved out of the way for clarity.

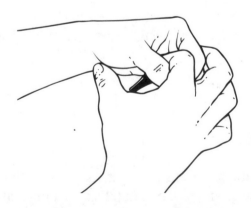

Diagram 42

You are actually stealing the speculum back into the right hand, where it is held by the thumb (this is a move known in magic as *palming*).

Keep the speculum hidden in your right palm, as shown in Diagram 43.

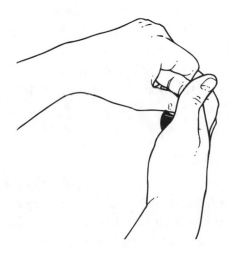

Diagram 43

Straighten out your right index finger and withdraw it from the loosely closed left fist. You will now act as if the speculum is in the left fist. Drop your right hand in a relaxed way to your side. Blow on the closed left fist and slowly open your left hand to display that the speculum has magically vanished.

Reach up to the patient's head with your right hand, and act as if you have found the speculum hiding behind his or her left ear. Your reaching motion must be such that the back of the right hand is always in the patient's view. This is to avoid having the child detect the speculum prematurely.

Once again repeat the same *Thimble Vanish*. But now when you reach up to the patient's ear, pretend to have trouble finding it. Tug a bit on the ear, asking the patient to turn his or her ear toward you. Squint a bit and grab your "magic light" (otoscope) to get a better look. Make the search (exam) funny—act puzzled, and talk to the speculum. *"Where did you go, you little rascal?"* Then quickly search the other ear. *"Not here."* Examine the nose. *"Not in there."* Examine the mouth. *"Where could you be hiding?"* Just as you finish with the patient's mouth, look surprised as you stare directly at your magic light (otoscope). Act shocked and a little embarrassed to find the speculum on the end of your otoscope, *"It's been right here in front of me all along!"*

PROFESSIONAL TIP:

Make sure that you straighten out your right index finger when you withdraw it from the left fist. If your finger is still curved, the illusion won't look right. Also relax your right hand when *palming*. The more relaxed and natural you appear, the more magical the trick will be. The focus of the illusion is to find the missing speculum. It is in this fun sequence of searching that you actually perform your ENT exam.

Make sure to set a new speculum onto the otoscope after the exam. We suggest that you do this in front of the parent and/or patient. This will set their minds at ease regarding the use of sterile equipment. After doing this a few times, it simply becomes procedure.

You might begin by introducing the speculum as a hat for your finger. Then, once it has vanished, explain that you are looking for your finger hat.

If you have trouble securing the speculum on your index finger, try slightly moistening it prior to performance. A quick dab on your index finger and you're good to go. Do this surreptitiously, when the patient is not looking.

. . . .

"This trick looks like it is difficult to learn. But the kids go silent and stare with their mouths open... I just love that."

Ellen Rabun, M.D.
Blacksburg, VA

. . . .

The Hat That Got Fat

🖊 Familiarization with a medical device

⊛ Examination aid

⧗ Time-saver

① Skill level

PREVIEW:

This is an alternative to the previous effect. It is ideal when a larger (surgical or sterilized) speculum is needed.

Fx:

Referring to your disposable speculum as a hat for your finger, you make it double in size right before the patient's eyes.

EXPLANATION:

Begin with the larger speculum in your left pocket. Place the smaller one in your right pocket.

When ready to perform, reach into each pocket with the appropriate hand. While doing so, ask the patient if he or she has ever seen a finger hat. About the time you receive a negative reply, bring out both hands.

The larger speculum is hidden in the curled left fingers as you focus the child's attention on the smaller speculum in the right hand. Make sure the wider end of each specula (the end that attaches to the otoscope) is facing the index finger and thumb.

Do not make a fist around the larger speculum in the left hand. Rather, keep the fingers lightly curled around it, as shown in Diagram 44.

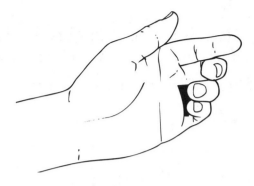

Diagram 44

As you explain that the smaller speculum is a hat for your fin-ger, jostle the fingers into position and slide the speculum onto your index finger, as shown in Diagram 45.

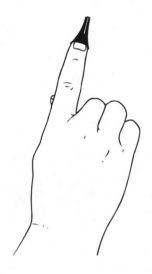

Diagram 45

Now it is okay to close the left hand into a tighter fist as you place the right index finger into the left hand. As you do, sim-ply slide the small speculum into the larger one. There may be a small noise here as the plastic makes contact. Simply adjust your patter, and you can easily cover it with the volume of your speech. This action is illustrated in Diagram 46. However, the left-hand fingers are shown loosened to facilitate your view. In practice, they will be closed, as shown in Diagram 47.

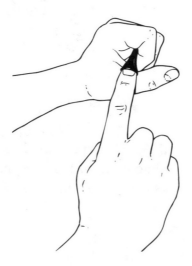

Diagram 46

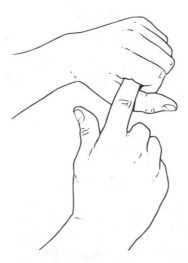

Diagram 47

Now when you remove your left hand, the spectator will see an enlarged speculum, as shown in Diagram 48. Notice the difference in speculum size between this diagram and Diagram 45.

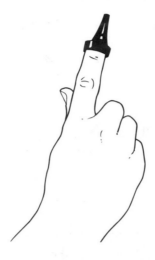

Diagram 48

The small speculum is hidden by virtue of being nested into the larger one. Explain that your *"Hat Got Fat."*

PROFESSIONAL TIP:

You'll need what magicians call a *clean up* to dispose of the smaller speculum. With the left hand, remove both specula as one from your right fingertip. To accomplish this, make sure your left thumb covers the opening to prevent the small speculum from falling out or just place your finger into your pocket to dispose of both specula.

Here, There, Nowhere, Everywhere

✖   Rapport builder

➤   Familiarization with a medical device

⊕   Examination aid

⧗   Time-saver

④   Skill level

PREVIEW:

This takes the *palming* move you mastered in the last two effects to a higher level. As a result, it requires additional practice. In order to master this piece, it will require about an hour of your time.

Fx:

The speculum from your otoscope (also known as your *Finger Hat*) takes an impressive journey. It appears, disappears, and even jumps from one finger to the other.

EXPLANATION:

Begin by introducing the speculum, telling the child that it is a hat for your finger. Proceed to cover your right-hand index finger with the speculum, as outlined in Diagram 45 of the previous effect *(The Hat That Got Fat)*.

Now, continuing with the previous set of moves, insert the speculum into the left hand, as shown in Diagram 47 of the previous effect. Steal the speculum just as you did earlier in *The 45-Second ENT Exam*. This steal was covered in Diagrams 42 and 43. Complete the disappearance according to the instructions at the beginning of *The 45-Second ENT Exam*, by *palming* the speculum in the right hand and showing your left hand empty.

Thus far you have duplicated the first part of the effects you have already learned. Here's where it goes to the next level. Insert your right middle finger into the left hand. Your hands should look like the illustration in Diagram 49. Notice that the *palmed* speculum is hidden from view. However, it is actually squeezed between the palm and the base of the thumb.

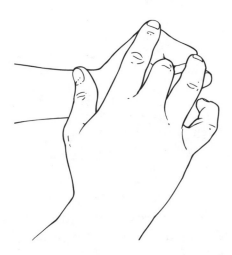

Diagram 49

Now, under cover of the left hand, the right hand's second finger reaches through the hand and steals the speculum from the right hand palm by inserting the fingertip into the opening of the speculum and onto the right middle fingertip. This is the same retrieval action you did earlier. This is shown from behind in Diagram 50.

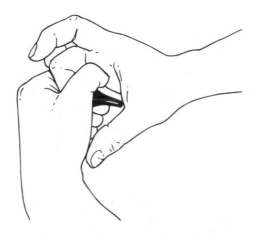

Diagram 50

Once you've secured the speculum on your right middle finger, straighten it within the left hand. Now remove the left-hand cover by pulling it up and away from the right hand. This will expose the speculum sitting on the right middle fingertip, as shown in Diagram 51.

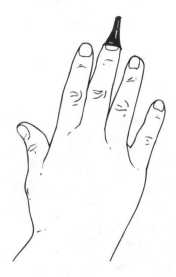

Diagram 51

PROFESSIONAL TIP:

It is important to move the left hand away from the right rather than to pull the right hand out from the left. This is because you don't want to dislodge the speculum, which is more likely to happen when removing the right hand, as opposed to the left. It should all happen very quickly.

Ultimate Speculum Magic

✖ Rapport builder

✐ Familiarization with a medical device

⊕ Examination aid

⏳ Time-saver

⑤ Skill level

PREVIEW:

There is no simple way around it—this will require significant practice. But it is the most visual piece of amazement in the book. If you've mastered the previous effect, you will soon dismiss it for this piece. We just didn't want to give you everything at once, so as not to overwhelm you.

This needs to be done very quickly in order to achieve maximum effect for the spectator. In addition, you may be unable to perform this if all your fingers do not adhere well to the plastic of the speculum. Adding moisturizer or hand lotion may not solve the adherence problem. However, if you have fingers that hold fast to the article, and you're willing to invest some time to practice, this will undoubtedly become one of your favorites.

It ranks high as a rapport builder. The child's eyes will pop from their sockets as he or she watches your wizardry in action.

Fx:

Your speculum (*Finger Hat*) jumps from one fingertip to the other with the simple flick of your hand.

EXPLANATION:

Begin with the speculum on your right index fingertip. Notice in Diagram 52 that all the fingers are extended. The back of your hand should face the patient.

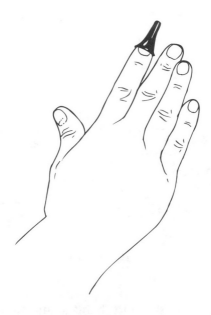

Diagram 52

Here's where things get difficult. Close the fingers and deposit the speculum into the right thumb *palm position* you learned earlier. Immediately—and we mean immediately—extend the fingers back to where they were. Diagram 53 shows your position (an exposed position) after the move is completed. Remember, the spectator sees the back of your hand, as shown in Diagram 54, with the speculum hidden from view.

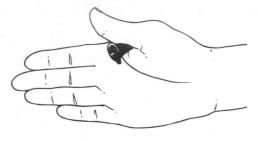

Diagram 53

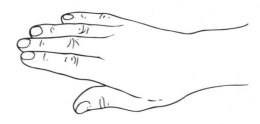

Diagram 54

Without pause, close the right hand again. Secure the speculum on the middle finger as shown in Diagram 55, and immediately extend all your fingers. Your position will be like that shown in Diagram 56.

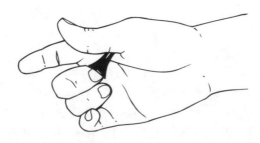

Diagram 55

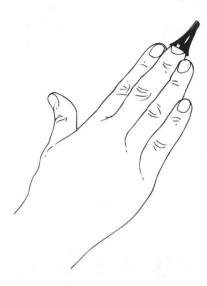

Diagram 56

Continue by again closing the fingers and depositing the speculum back into *palming* position and immediately extend the fingers. Now the fingers bend again, and the ring finger grabs the speculum. Once more, extend your fingers. If you're still with us, your position should be like that shown in Diagram 57.

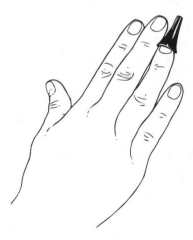

Diagram 57

Finally, close the hands again and allow the ring finger to leave the device in thumb palm. Open the fingers to show it gone, and immediately close them so the baby finger can steal the *Finger Hat.*

You've done it. Your final position should be like that shown in Diagram 58.

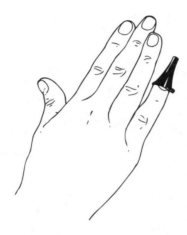

Diagram 58

PROFESSIONAL TIP:

The whole exercise should take no more than five seconds to complete. Some doctors have told us that this is an excellent numbers review for prekindergarteners to measure their counting skills.

Skillful Swabs

Those culture sticks can provide an ideal solution not only for engaging the patient but also occupying them during exam room waiting time.

Curious Swab Game

✎ Familiarization with a medical device

🎲 Game

🗨 Clinical reasoning and thinking assessment

⧗ Time-saver

① Skill level

PREVIEW:

The beauty of this effect is that it is not only quick but also easy to do.

YOU'LL NEED:

Four swabs. You will also need a coin or other round object. You can even use the speculum from your otoscope. Many physicians are now using antimicrobial diaphragms for their stethoscopes. Again, any small round object will do.

FX:

We recommend that this be used as a puzzle to keep the patient busy after being placed in the examining room and awaiting

---

the doctor's entrance. It serves to absorb the patient's mind and thereby remove the anxiety that accompanies those several minutes of waiting in a daunting environment.

While taking the patient's vital signs, have your M.A. or nurse explain this puzzle in advance of your entrance. When you walk in, you can solve the puzzle in less than one second. It's a perfect lead-in to solving the real puzzle of the patient's illness.

Have the four swabs set up as shown in Diagram 59, placing the coin *inside* the U-shaped center. You can explain that it is a glass of soda with a cherry in it. Or for football fans, say it is the ball going through the goal posts.

We recommend using the small-size cotton-tipped applicators and setting up the enigma on the examining table.

The object is for the patient to move ONLY TWO swabs in such a way that the cherry is outside of the glass, as shown in Diagram 60.

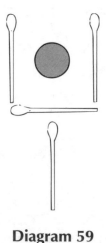

Diagram 59

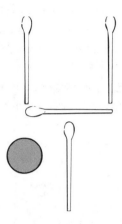

Diagram 60

EXPLANATION:

The secret to success is very simple, once you know it. Note Diagram 61. Begin by sliding Swab C halfway, until it is perpendicular to Swab A, essentially forming an upside down T. (You can see how this should look by examining Diagram 62, noting the positions of Swabs A and C.)

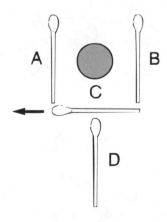

Diagram 61

Then bring Swab B down to the end of C, as shown in Diagram 62.

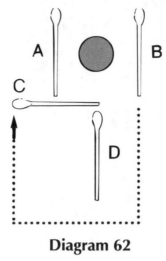

Diagram 62

The result is shown in Diagram 63.

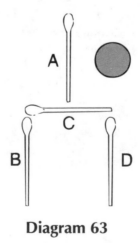

Diagram 63

PROFESSIONAL TIP:

If your assistant has properly set up the game, all you have to do is enter the room and solve the problem at the drop of a dime.

Vanishing Swab

✖   Rapport builder

↗   Familiarization with a medical device

⊕   Examination aid

⌛   Time-saver

①   Skill level

PREVIEW:

You can have a lot of fun with this, and the child will love you because you let him or her in on the secret. It's a very fast way to break the ice with even the most distant and introverted patient. You'll need a long cotton-tipped applicator and a cotton ball. You'll find this effect a perfect solution when you need a throat culture or strep screen.

Fx:

While explaining to the child that you can make the cotton ball disappear, you inadvertently make the swab disappear. Then, showing the secret of where the swab went, you refocus your attention on the cotton ball, only to find that it has, indeed, vanished.

EXPLANATION:

The patient should be to your left side. Begin with a cotton ball in your left hand. You may want to store the swab in your breast pocket for easy access.

Show the cotton ball and explain that you have a magic stick, just like magicians have magic wands. Inform the patient that your magic stick will make the cotton ball disappear, simply by

---

tapping it three times. Remove the swab from your breast pocket and use it to point to the cotton ball, as shown in Diagram 64.

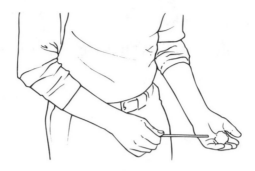

Diagram 64

Ask the child to help you count to three. *"One, Two, Three."* With each number swing the swab upward then back down. Bring it up high, near the side of your face, as you count *"One."* When you count *"Two,"* bring it higher still, until it is near your temple. When you reach *"Three,"* the swab should be up past your ear as depicted in Diagram 65.

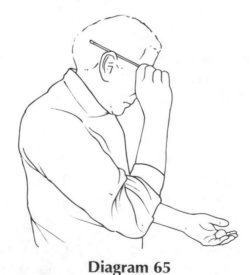

Diagram 65

When you reach *"Three,"* leave the swab behind your right ear, as shown in Diagram 66. But without missing a beat, bring the empty right hand down to the left.

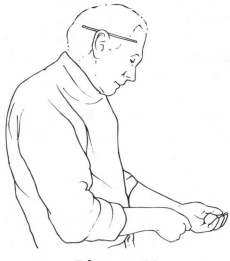

Diagram 66

Say, *"Oh no. I think that instead of the cotton ball disappearing, the magic stick disappeared."*

Clearly show your hands, as illustrated in Diagram 67.

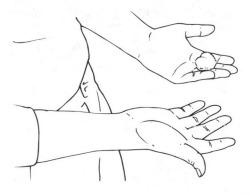

Diagram 67

Now you'll expose where the swab went. Turn your body so that your right ear is facing the patient and point to the swab with your right index finger.

Here's the kicker. With your left side now away from the patient, drop the cotton ball into the left outside pocket of your lab coat or pants. Showing the swab behind your ear provides perfect cover for this subterfuge.

Once the gag registers in the child's mind, turn back to fully face him or her and say, *"Now, where did the cotton ball go?"* Show both hands empty.

PROFESSIONAL TIP:

This is an excellent piece that requires only a few minute's practice. It is a simple matter of timing your turns. Best of all, it introduces the child to both medical devices in a fun way, and in addition you've broken through any barriers the child may have erected.

· ·

"This book is just what the doctor ordered. After using a few of these tricks on our pediatric ambulatory emergency department patients, I found it much easier to examine and treat the patient. I'm sure it will have a positive impact on our patient satisfaction scores."

Dennis Guest, D.O., F.A.C.O.E.P., F.A.C.E.P.
Chairman, Emergency Department
Northeastern Hospital
Philadelphia, PA

· ·

It Floats

✎ Familiarization with a medical device

⚕ Examination aid

⧖ Time-saver

② Skill level

PREVIEW:

To start, we recommend that you keep a swab in your breast pocket. This is another time-saver that will motivate the patient to think about how you made that giant swab float, thereby alleviating his or her tension regarding the upcoming exam.

FX:

As you just read, a culture stick seems to float behind your hand while all fingers are apparently showing.

EXPLANATION:

The key to the explanation lies in the term *apparently.* It will look as if all your fingers are showing, but in reality that is not the case. But we are putting the cart before the horse. Let's look at it step by step. You should stand directly facing the child.

Begin by pointing your fingertips together, as shown in Diagram 68.

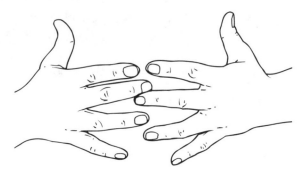

Diagram 68

Now dovetail your fingers together such that the middle fingers enter the palm of the opposite hand, as shown in Diagram 69.

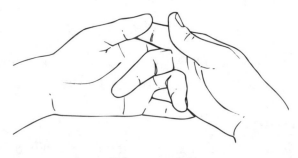

Diagram 69

We should issue a word of warning here. This is a very simple movement. However, it is also unnatural. Your brain will want to place your right third and fourth fingers over the third and fourth fingers of the left hand. You have to be conscious of this and force your mind to overcome its natural tendency. Practicing for about fifteen minutes easily accomplishes this.

When done correctly, the outside of your hands (the patient's view) will look exactly as shown in Diagram 70. Notice how all the fingers appear to be showing. However, from your view (Diagram 69), the two middle fingers are hidden behind the scenes. Again, after a few minutes of practice, you can complete this task as if it were second nature.

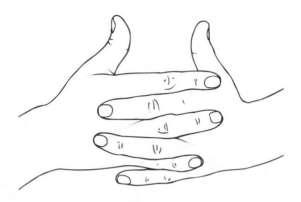

Diagram 70

Once you have this move down pat, you can proceed to the next portion of the effect. You will notice that the two middle fingers can operate rather freely as they hide behind your palms. This will be a necessary function, as you are about to see.

With the hands properly dovetailed, bring them up to your breast pocket. As you move your hands upward and toward the culture stick, say to the child, *"Watch. I'm going to make that stick float right out of my pocket."* Allow the two middle fingers to grasp the swab, and then move them away from your body and towards the patient. From the child's perspective, your position will be like that shown in Diagram 71.

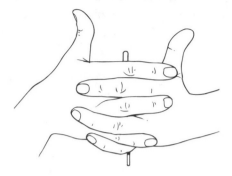

Diagram 71

Ask the patient to hold out his or her hands in a cup position. Now situate your own hands over the patient's hands and release the grasp held by your two middle fingers, allowing the swab to fall into the child's waiting hands.

Open your hands to show that they are empty.

PROFESSIONAL TIP:

Present the swab to the patient as a gift. Tell him or her to go home and practice and to let you know on the next return visit how he or she made out. By now the swab is no big deal to the child, and you are set to proceed with your exam. Plus, he or she may even be excited about the return visit.

One doctor recommended using this on an impacted earwax patient. He follows with a warning to never place a cotton-tipped swab fully into the ear canal.

Speaking of warnings…*Small object warning! Only give this to the patient as a souvenir when age appropriate.*

Here are a few more puzzles. These can be done by lining up a few swabs according to the diagrams below.

Swab Swami

✗   Rapport builder

⚅   Game

🗨   Clinical reasoning and thinking assessment

①   Skill level

. . . .

You will find the answers to these riddles on Page 207.

. . . .

1) Lay six swabs on the table as indicated in Diagram 72. Ask the patient to add five more swabs and make them equal only nine.

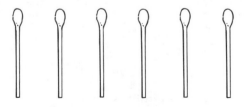

Diagram 72

2) Ask the patient to lay six swabs on the table (without breaking them) and make them equal to three and a half dozen.

3) Lay four swabs on the table as indicated in Diagram 73, and ask the patient to make it ten by adding only five more swabs.

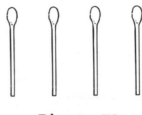

Diagram 73

4) Ask the patient to lay down seven swabs (as shown in Diagram 74), remove one, and leave nothing.

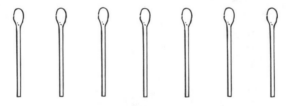

Diagram 74

5) Hand the patient five swabs and ask if he or she can make two triangles (without bending or breaking the swabs).

6) Give the patient nine swabs and ask if he or she can make them into five triangles (without bending or breaking the swabs).

. . . .

"These magic effects are an excellent distraction for the waiting patient. They stimulate the mind while keeping the patient unaware of the passing time."

Alicia Bednar, R.N.
West Hills, CA

. . . .

Glove Magic

Dime through Glove

- ✂ Rapport builder
- ✎ Familiarization with a medical device
- ① Skill level

PREVIEW:

This is one of the most visually stunning effects in the entire book. It allows for one-on-one, patient/doctor rapport building. It's a hands-on experience for the patient (who really does feel the dime go through the glove). And it's unbelievably simple to learn! After reading the explanation, you'll be performing this effect almost immediately!

FX:

A dime magically penetrates through a solid and uncompromised rubber exam glove. Once the effect is completed, the glove and the dime can be thoroughly examined by the patient. There is no fear of exposing the magical "secret."

EXPLANATION:

This trick requires latex exam gloves (preferably nonpowdered). Currently many physicians are concerned about latex allergies and reactions. If this is a concern in your practice, please continue to use your vinyl gloves for your day-to-day exams. However, this ploy specifically takes advantage of the particular properties of latex, and vinyl gloves simply will not work. It is such a good effect that you may want to keep a box of latex gloves handy to use only for performances.

Have a close look at Diagram 75. A dime only appears to be resting on the palm of the latex glove. In actuality, the dime is inside the glove the entire time! The latex rubber is pushed up from the inside, and the rubber is tightly stretched around the dime.

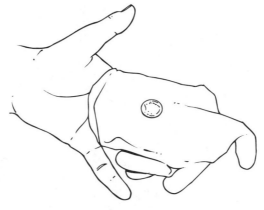

Diagram 75

Here's the secret. The best way to position the dime is to place it atop a magic marker or a thick highlighter pen, as shown in Diagram 76.

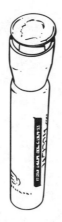

Diagram 76

Stretch the glove, placing the inside portion of the glove's palm over the coin. Now push downward, as shown in Diagram 77.

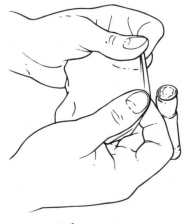

Diagram 77

Latex rubber, when stretched almost to the breaking point, appears to be clear or transparent. By pushing the dime up from the inside, the latex "grips" and contracts around the edges of the coin (see Diagram 78), causing it to have an incredible 3-D-like appearance from the other side.

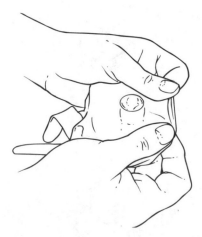

Diagram 78

When you feel that the dime is secured by the grip of the latex, gently lift it from the magic marker. (Once you become proficient at it, you will be able to load the dime freehand, without need of a marker.)

Chances are, while rehearsing this effect, you'll break or pop several gloves. This is normal. Don't worry. You'll find the right tension, and you'll soon be pushing the dime into position without any trouble.

Carefully place your fingers into the glove to obtain a position similar to that shown in Diagram 79. Once you have it down pat, you can use the patient's hand, inserting it into the glove, and enhancing his or her perception of penetration.

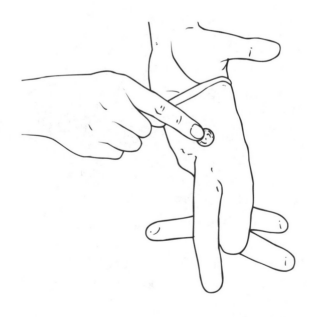

Diagram 79

When the dime is pushed down from the outside of the glove, the rubber snaps back to its original, relaxed state. It is this "snap" that makes it *feel* like the dime has gone right through the glove.

Display the glove to the patient and ask him or her to use the pointer finger to push down on the dime, as illustrated in Diagram 79. As this is done, the dime will magically disappear from view and "snap" through the glove and into the patient's waiting hand. See Diagram 80. The dime has disappeared from view and penetrated the glove.

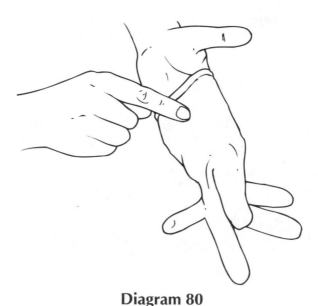

Diagram 80

Slowly slide the glove off the fingers to reveal the dime, as shown in Diagram 81, strengthening the visual effect to the onlooker.

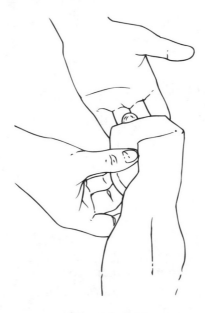

Diagram 81

Allow the patient to examine the glove and the dime as you ask him or her to try to find the hole.

PROFESSIONAL TIP:

You can make several of these "prepared" gloves ahead of time and keep them in the top drawer of your cabinet for use throughout the day. It is also a wonderful idea for your hospital rounds!

Caution! Popped balloons are the number-one choking object for small children. Remember, only give a glove or balloon to an age-appropriate child.

Happy Face

✖ Rapport Builder

➤ Familiarization with a medical device

③ Skill level

PREFACE:

Have you ever blown up an exam glove and given it to a child as a balloon? This is always an old standby that many health-care workers learn early on in their residency. But there must be a better way, or a more "engaging" way, to present this make-shift balloon to the patient.

Fx:

Simply take a magic marker and either write the patient's name on the glove, or draw a happy face. The number-one concern is that the patient is NOT allergic to latex.

EXPLANATION:

Blow up a glove, tie it off, and go to town.

PROFESSIONAL TIP:

Around Thanksgiving, try making the glove into a turkey to add to the festivities.

The Dreaded Needle
(Needle through Glove)

✖ Rapport builder

💉 Familiarization with a medical device

② Skill level

PREFACE:

Many health-care workers have asked us for an effect with a needle. Most likely, an injection is the number-one tension builder during any child's office visit. Most children have learned from an early age that shots can hurt or be scary!

In certain instances, it may help to familiarize the patient with the needle to help make the inoculation less traumatic. If you happen to find yourself in this situation, the *needle through the glove* effect might be the perfect trick to add to your repertoire.

FX:

An exam glove is blown up and tied off like a balloon. A happy face is then drawn on the glove. Once this is done, a needle is jabbed into the glove without causing the glove to pop or deflate.

EXPLANATION:

There are two ways to perform this effect. Each method has its pros and cons. In both methods, once completed, the glove must be discarded quickly, due to the fact that the air will eventually escape from the small hole, causing the glove to deflate.

Method 1:

Stick a small one-inch piece of scotch tape onto an already inflated glove. When you enter the room, simply start by drawing a happy face on one side of the glove. We've found that a permanent pen such as a Magic Marker or a Sharpie works best. Keep the taped spot of the glove turned away from the patient. If you stick a needle into the tape, the glove will not pop (see Diagram 82). If you have difficulty tying off a glove, you may try using scotch tape to tightly wrap it, in lieu of an actual knot.

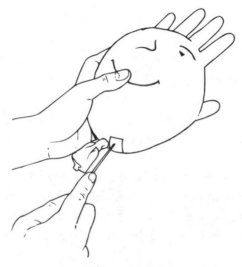

Diagram 82

The advantage to this method is a near 100 percent success rate in keeping the glove from popping. The disadvantage is that the child can't directly see the injection site (because he or she would clearly see the tape and discover your secret).

Method 2:

Start by preparing a needle with a light coat of KY jelly. Inflate the glove so that it is full of air, but don't stretch the glove to its breaking point. The idea here is to add just enough air so that the glove looks inflated, without making it too "tight." Draw a happy face on the glove and pick up the needle. Look carefully at the glove in its inflated state. You'll notice that there is a difference in the thickness of the "skin" of the glove from one area to another. You will probably notice that the palm of the glove is the weakest and thinnest point in the glove, while the fingertips have the thickest and strongest surface. Obviously, to keep the glove from popping, we'll insert the needle in the thickest area of the glove. The KY jelly on the needle performs two important functions. First, it lubricates the entry point of the needle and keeps the glove from tearing. Second, it helps to form an air-tight seal in the glove while the needle is inserted. And that is all there is to it! Just be careful with your touch with this method. If you are too forceful, the glove may pop, having the opposite effect on your patient than the one you desire. The advantage with this method is that the injection point can be shown up close, without fear of the patient discovering the secret!

PATTER:

"I understand that you are a little worried about today's vaccination. Did you know that at one time I was afraid of vacations too? Oh, sure, vacations can be a little scary unless you know about my friend Gobble the Glove." Blow up a glove and draw a picture of a turkey instead of the happy face shown above.

"His least favorite vacation was always thanksgiving. Oh, excuse me, you were worried about a vaccination not a vacation. That's not a problem for my friend Gobble here. Look, he's a balloon, and did you know that a balloon's number-one enemy is always a needle? You would think that a needle would pop a balloon like this, wouldn't you? But with my help and expertise, even Gobble the Glove is safe from harm. Just watch." Put the needle into the glove without popping it. *"See, if Gobble can do it, so can you! And if you begin to get scared or feel like*

you want to cry, just make the sound of a turkey. Say, 'gobble-gobble,' and it'll be over before you know it!"

PROFESSIONAL TIP:

Once you remove the needle (in either method) the air will begin to escape on its own. Throw the glove away immediately, toss it out the door, or pop it in some other way to keep your secret safe!

· ·

A Note about the Federal Needlestick Safety and Prevention Act, November 2000.

As of this printing of *Side-Fx*, there are over 207 separate needlestick safety devices produced by over 90 different companies. Obviously, it is difficult for the authors to experiment with each device to insure their success in effects described. As with all magic, please practice the effect before performing it in front of a live audience.

And remember, it is always important to perform these effects with an unused, clean needle, to avoid any possible needlestick injuries to the health-care provider or patient.

For more information on needlestick safety and a list of current OSHA-approved devices, please visit http://www.healthsystem.virginia.edu/internet/epinet/ or contact:

International Health-care Worker Safety Center
University of Virginia
P.O. Box 800764
Charlottesville, VA 22908-0764
(434) 924-5159

· ·

Miscellaneous Examining Room Items

L isted here are effects that require a few more items that can
be found in the examining room.

The Hammer Knows

✷   Rapport builder

✐   Familiarization with a medical device

☑   You've just done the exam

⊕   Examination aid

🐾   Clinical motor skill experiment

⧗   Time-saver

①   Skill level

PREVIEW:

Since it is imperative for the child to be completely relaxed
during reflex testing, this is an ideal effect to avoid that "knee-
jerk" reaction (pun intended) when the child first sees the
hammer. It is fun, and familiarizes the patient with the medical
device.

The effect will require a small amount of advance preparation.
But once completed, you will be set for all your future performances.

To begin, take four 3x5-inch index cards. Using a magic marker, number the blank side of each card with numbers 1 through 4. See Diagram 83.

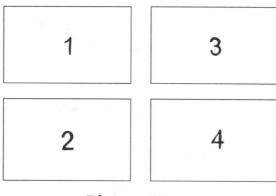

Diagram 83

After the cards are numbered, turn them over, placing the numbers face down. Using a pencil, you will place small marks on the front of the four cards. This is the side with preprinted lines. These marks will tell you the number on the other side of the card.

CARD MARKED #1:

Place a small pencil dot on each edge of the card on its short sides, at about the center. Again, this is on the reverse side of where the number "1" is. Diagram 84 shows an exaggerated mark. In practice, you'll want to make this mark as lightly as possible, so it will be recognizable to you, but not so to anyone else.

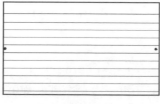

Diagram 84

CARD MARKED #2:

Place a small pencil mark *(very lightly)*, on the diagonal corners of the card. See Diagram 85.

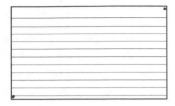

Diagram 85

CARD MARKED #3:

Place a small pencil mark *(very lightly)*, at the approximate center of each of the long sides of the card, as shown in Diagram 86.

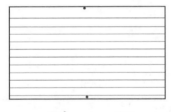

Diagram 86

CARD MARKED #4:

No marks are made to this card. It remains blank, as shown in Diagram 87.

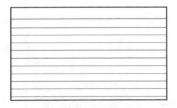

Diagram 87

If you prefer, you could buy a pack of "Uno" cards and mark the backs as indicated above.

Fx:

After handing the patient all four cards, tell him or her to mix them up and remove one. Have the child look at the card and remember the number that appears on it. Explain that your magic hammer will tell you which number was removed. Sure enough, your reflex hammer gives a clear indication of the selected number to both the practitioner and the patient.

EXPLANATION:

Assuming the child removed the card marked #3, begin the exam, but DO NOT tap the patellar tendon. Rather, tap *away* from it, so as NOT to elicit a reflex response. Say, *"Number One."*

Repeat the procedure a second time, same as before. Except this time you will say, *"Number Two."*

On the third rap, you will actually tap the patellar tendon as you say, *"Number Three."* When you have observed the patellar reflex and recorded the DTR, announce, *"Aha. You had the card marked Number Three. My magic hammer never misses."*

Not only did you amaze the patient, but you were also able to make an evaluation relative to the child's nervous system. The child is left wondering how your magic hammer knew the number, and is not thinking one iota about the exam.

PROFESSIONAL TIP:

You can save lots of time by having your nurse or M.A. do the prework in advance. When she leaves the examining room, she can leave a post-it note on the chart, telling you the number the child selected. Then all you have to do is the magic when you do the exam.

The Singing Magic Gizmo

�   Rapport builder

✐   Familiarization with a medical device

☑   You've just done the exam

⊕   Examination aid

⧗   Time-saver

①   Skill level

PREVIEW:

You'll find this an ideal way to relax the child, make him or her smile, and complete an audiology exam, all at the same time. If you need to evaluate proprioception or perform a Rinne or Weber Test, the minor preparation needed will be well worth the effort. As with the previous piece, you may want your nurse or M.A. to take care of the preselection process in advance.

If you read the last effect, you'll find that this is really the same dodge. However, instead of using numbers you'll use colors.

Fx:

Show the child four index cards. Each has a different color on one side. After handing the patient all four cards, tell the child to remove the one that has his or her favorite color.

After introducing your singing magic gizmo (the tuning fork), explain that it will sing when you name the child's favorite color (which he or she previously removed from the stack of cards). As with the reflex hammer, your instrument proves to be correct.

EXPLANATION:

The method is the same as for the previous effect, with minor variations.

To begin, take four 3x5-inch index cards. Instead of using numbers, use a crayon to draw a smiley face on the blank side of each card, using a different color for each card.

Card #1 – Draw a RED smiley

Card #2 – Draw a BLUE smiley

Card #3 – Draw a GREEN smiley

Card #4 – Draw a YELLOW smiley

After the faces have been drawn, turn the cards over, placing the drawings face down. Using a pencil, place the small marks on the back of each card, as follows.

CARD WITH RED SMILEY:

Place a small pencil mark *(very lightly)* on each edge of the card on its short sides, at about the center. (Refer to Diagram 84 in the previous effect.)

CARD WITH BLUE SMILEY:

Place a small pencil mark *(very lightly)* on the diagonal corners of the card. (Refer to Diagram 85 in the previous effect.)

CARD WITH GREEN SMILEY:

Place a small pencil mark *(very lightly)* at the approximate center of each of the long sides of the card. (Refer to Diagram 86 in the previous effect.)

CARD WITH YELLOW SMILEY:

No marks are made to this card. It remains blank. (Refer to Diagram 87 in the previous effect.)

To perform, take the cards between your hands and show the different colored faces. Then turn them facing down (the marked side up). Have the child remove one of the smiley faces. As the card is removed, look at the back to determine which one was taken. It's that simple. The rest is all byplay.

Explain that you have a "Singing Magic Gizmo" that will tell you which color the child removed. Introduce the tuning fork and mention that the "Gizmo" always sings when you mention the color that was chosen.

Let's assume the child chose the card with the Green smiley. Take the tuning fork in your right hand and tap it against the left index finger, as illustrated in Diagram 88. (If you're used to tapping it against your elbow, you may have to make an alteration and use your left hand.) Notice the spot at which the left finger contacts the tuning fork. It is at the base of the element. Thus, no sound will emit from the instrument.

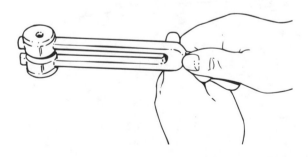

Diagram 88

As you do so, ask the tuning fork. *"Did my friend take the red face?"*

Raise the tuning fork to the child's ear and ask if he or she can hear the Magic Gizmo sing. Now, because no sound comes from the fork, explain that he or she did not choose red. Explain that if red had been chosen, the tuning fork would sing its song. Continue as before.

"Did my friend choose yellow?" As you say this, strike the tuning fork again, exactly as before. Again, lift the tuning fork to the child's ear and ask if the Gizmo is singing.

"Hmmm. You did not choose yellow either. Let's try again."

Say, *"Did my friend choose green?"*

This time, strike the fork as you would to make it reverberate—at a higher point of the element, as illustrated in Diagram 89.

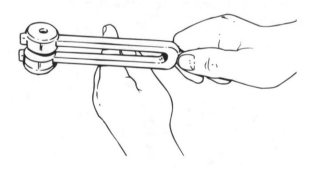

Diagram 89

When you raise the tuning fork to the patient's ear, he or she will hear its humming sound and the child's eyes will widen in awe.

Say, " *Aha. You chose the green, and that's why the Singing Gizmo is singing its song.*"

PROFESSIONAL TIP:

You can easily use this method to do either a Rinne or Weber Test. All you do is shift the location of the tuning fork from the ear to the Mastoid process, depending on your test. In either case, you will have examined the child before he or she knows it.

Instead of drawing marks on the index cards, you could cut a tiny tip from the corner of a card. Another card can have two corners cut, and so on.

Several doctors mentioned that this is a great idea for kids with tubes in their eardrums. *"I can sometimes see through your ear to the other side."* Have the child hold the selected card to the opposite ear being examined. The patient will be concentrating on holding the card next to his or her ear. The physician announces that he can see the color through the other side.

Cut and Restored Stethoscope

✖ Rapport builder

✎ Familiarization with a medical device

⑤ Skill level

PREFACE:

This effect is a wonderful grand finale, as you say a happy good-bye to a long-term care patient...or you may want to use it as an excellent opener for your next speech. Technically it is not that hard to do, but the preparation time will prohibit you from performing it on a regular basis. However, under the right conditions this effect will make you a "real" magician, and we believe you will find it well worth the effort.

FX:

The "magician" cuts the tube on his stethoscope in half! He then clearly displays both ends and magically restores the stethoscope to its previously uncut status. The stethoscope can be freely used, examined, and handled before and after the effect! You can even borrow a colleague's stethoscope and use it for the presentation.

EXPLANATION:

Once again, this is a "special" effect that will take time to set up each time you perform it, but it is well worth the labor.

You'll need the following items:

• A stethoscope

• A lab coat or suit jacket

- A pair of scissors
- A safety pin
- Some round sewing elastic (available from any craft shop or Wal-Mart). Use white elastic if you will be wearing a lab coat or black elastic for a suit jacket.
- Heat-shrink tubing to match the color of your stethoscope (available at any Radio Shack as part number 278-1610 for red, white, or blue, or part number 278-1627 for black).

Cut a piece of the round elastic to about 18 to 24 inches in length. Tie one end of the elastic to the safety pin, and attach the pin to the inside of your coat or jacket. Pin it in the center of the coat at the seam in the back, just below your shoulder blades. Take a 6-inch piece of heat-shrink tubing and fold it in half. Take the two ends of the tubing and tie them to the other end of the elastic that is secured in your coat. To facilitate this tying action, you may want to take a sharp object like an ice pick and puncture the tubing. Then thread it with the elastic and tie it off. When finished, your coat should look similar to the one shown in Diagram 90.

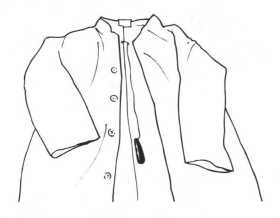

Diagram 90

We suggest using a length between 18 and 24 inches of elastic—the specific length depends on the size of the lab coat. Ideally you want the device to hang such that it is not exposed at the bottom of the coat. It should comfortably hang to your lower back at the belt line.

Put your lab coat on and let the elastic/tubing simply hang down your back inside the jacket. With your left hand, secretly reach around your back and grasp the tubing so that the folded end is pointing "up" in your hand, as shown in Diagram 91.

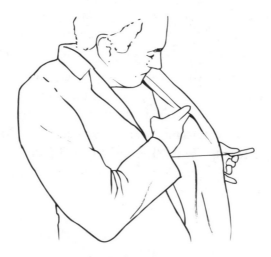

Diagram 91

Diagram 91 shows the tube in the hand, with the elastic running along the arm into the jacket.

If you take the stethoscope in your right hand and fold the tube in half, you'll notice that it looks just like our previously prepared piece of heat-shrink tubing. Transfer the folded stethoscope to your left hand. The fold of the actual stethoscope is kept down in the palm of your hand and the folded heat-shrink tubing is now displayed as if it were a real piece of the stethoscope. This is shown with an exposed view in Diagram 92.

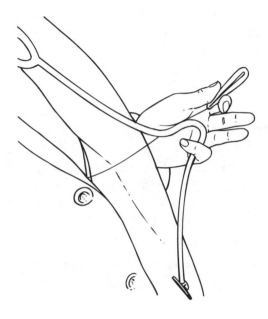

Diagram 92

Your left hand is now holding the real stethoscope (folded in half) in the palm, and the loop of heat-shrink tubing can clearly be seen extending from your fist. Pick up a pair of scissors in your right hand and simply cut the heat-shrink tubing loop in your left hand. Allow this moment to sink in to your viewer's consciousness. Clearly display the cut ends of the heat-shrink tubing.

At this point, if you loosen your grip on the heat-shrink tubing, you'll notice that the elastic will eject the tubing into your coat and behind your back. The elastic "pull" will help you to get rid of the pieces of heat-shrink tubing in your left hand. The problem with this "vanish" of the tubing is that the snap of the elastic may make a pop-like sound, exposing the secret, and/or your jacket may move in an unusual way, exposing the effect. To prevent the exposure of your secret and to make this effect believable, you'll need to make a larger movement with your entire body and arms to help you cover the smaller movement of the snapping elastic.

The movement should look something like this: once the tubing is cut, bring the cut ends to your mouth and blow on them. At the same time, loosen your grip on the pieces and extend your arms fully to display the restored stethoscope. This action should be performed as a single, deliberate, flowing movement for maximum effect and cover.

Hold out the now-restored stethoscope for examination and accept your well-deserved applause! Congratulations, you are now an official physician magician!

PROFESSIONAL TIP:

Practice, practice, practice! Try the *pull vanish* several times in front of the mirror before you perform it for an audience. Timing is everything here. The more time you spend in rehearsal, the better the effect will appear. Also, you can add some shine to the heat-shrink tubing and make it look more like a stethoscope by dressing the tubing with a small amount of Armor-All.

Also, be aware that if you are doing any cutting that requires the use of scissors, such as bandages, you now have a nifty way to introduce them.

Dry Ice Magic

✖   Rapport builder

😊   Just for fun

🎲   Game

①   Skill level

PREVIEW:

Each month, when the frozen vaccines arrive, packed in dry ice, the entire office becomes a playground. With the addition of this mischievous substance, the possibilities for magic quickly become apparent.

. . . .

Warning: Dry ice is frozen carbon dioxide (CO_2 at -109.3° F) as opposed to regular ice (H_2O at 32° F). Unlike regular ice, dry ice doesn't melt—it sublimates (the process of going directly from a solid to a gas). Dry ice should only be handled by adults or with adult supervision. When handling dry ice, be sure to use cotton or leather gloves. Do not allow anyone to touch dry ice directly with bare hands because it can burn.

. . . .

Fx:

Most people are aware of several magical-looking stunts that can be accomplished with dry ice. By adding a small amount of dry ice to warm water, you can make a foggy witches brew, produce a low-level mist on the floor, and even (carefully) put some of the fog (not ice) in your mouth to blow smoke rings. Here are some additional fun ideas you can use when it's dry-ice day in your office.

EXAM GLOVES THAT INFLATE THEMSELVES:

Place a small amount of dry ice inside a latex glove and tie it securely. As the solid ice begins to turn into CO_2 gas, the glove will inflate by itself, magically.

SMOKING SOAP SERPENT:

Take a cup or a bucket and mix hand soap with water. Once mixed, add the dry ice. A foaming serpent of bubbles will grow out of the bucket. And all of the bubbles will be filled with smoke. Have your patient pop the bubbles and watch as they smoke when popped!

POPPING MEDICINE BOTTLE:

This fun (and often harebrained) activity vividly demonstrates dry ice "sublimation." Place a piece of dry ice into a plastic (non-childproof) medicine container (the type with a pop-off lid). No need to add water—just wait. The lid will pop off, and sometimes fly several yards. Be careful not to aim for anyone's eyes. (Also, be careful not to use a childproof lid. If the lid can't pop off easily, you have just made a dry-ice bomb instead!)

Singing Metal:

Press a warm quarter firmly against a chunk of dry ice. The coin will "scream" piercingly as the heat causes the dry ice to instantly turn to gas. The pressure of escaping CO_2 pushes the coin away from the dry ice, and without contact, the dry ice stops "sublimating." The quarter falls back into contact with the solid ice again, and the cycle repeats. This all happens so quickly that the metal vibrates, causing the singing or screaming sound you hear. Try this stunt with other metal items in your office to discover various results!

Floating Bubbles:

For this stunt you'll also need some toy bubble solution: Make a dry-ice fog in the sink by mixing it with warm water. Simply blow soap bubbles onto the fog to see them float and dance. Are the bubbles really floating in midair? Or are they floating in mid-carbon dioxide? Or are they floating somewhere in-between the air and the carbon dioxide? If you watch closely, you will see the bubbles getting larger...and eating other bubbles. While the bubble is there, you can watch it change colors, because as a bubble gets older and thinner, it becomes transparent on top. Soon it will be so thin it will pop.

. . . .

"I use dry ice. It has provided many happy and fascinated patients. Some have remembered the magic years later."

Elliot Weinstein, M.D., F.A.A.P
Montclair, CA

. . . .

The No Knot Gambit

✖ Rapport builder

🎈 Clinical reasoning and thinking assessment

② Skill level

PREFACE:

Although the items needed for this effect are not immediately found in the examining room, we couldn't resist giving you the opportunity to evaluate it.

This conundrum will have the child patient scratching his or her head. Additionally, you will get a peek at the patient's deductive skills. Add to this the fact that you will be building a relationship with the patient that will facilitate your examination, and you may find yourself running out to secure the items necessary to do the effect.

For this you will need a shoelace and a tube of some sort. Any hollow tubular device will do, even a cardboard tube from a toilet paper roll.

Fx:

After seemingly tying a knot around the tube and having the patient secure the ends of the tube, you cause the knot to disappear.

EXPLANATION:

Explain to the patient that the tube has magical properties. *"Here, I'll show you what I mean."*

Tie a single overhand knot around the outside of your tube. See Diagram 93. Then thread one end of the shoelace through the passageway of the tube, and ask the child patient to hold that end. Make sure to tell him or her not to pull, just to hold it firmly.

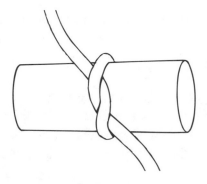

Diagram 93

Now slide the entire knot off the tube toward the same end where the string originally went through (opposite end that the patient is still holding). Bunch up the knot in your hand as it is removed from the tube, and pack the whole wad inside the tube. See Diagram 94.

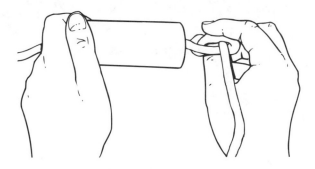

Diagram 94

Take the remaining shoelace end and have the patient hold it tightly in his or her free hand. Once the patient has secured both ends of the shoelace, begin moving the tube back and forth. The knot is gone, despite the fact that your patient is holding both ends of the shoelace.

The secret is effortless. You thread the end of the shoelace into the tube from *under* the knot. If you threaded it from over the knot, the knot would actually do the reverse and double.

Examine the figures below. Diagram 95 shows the underneath threading procedure, which will cause the knot to become undone. If you thread the shoelace over the top, as shown in Diagram 96, the trick will fail, and you will produce a double knot.

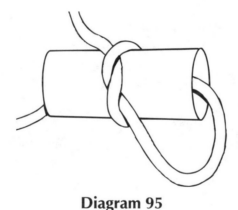

Diagram 95

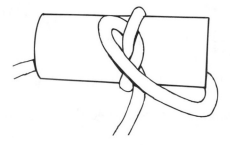

Diagram 96

PROFESSIONAL TIP:

You may want to let some patients attempt the feat. If so, tie the knot as in Diagram 96 and allow the trick to fail. It only works for you. Alternatively, you could tie the knot such that it comes off, allowing the child to succeed as well. We recommend the latter.

Leaping Band-Aid

✖ Rapport builder

🐾 Clinical motor skill experiment

🎗 Clinical reasoning and thinking assessment

⏳ Time-saver

① Skill level

PREVIEW:

This is an excellent time-saver. All you'll need to do is wrap a band-aid around your middle finger, at the base of the nail.

Fx:

A band-aid appears to jump from one finger to another. It all happens in the blink of an eye.

EXPLANATION:

Place a band-aid around your right middle finger, as shown in Diagram 97.

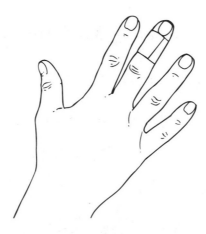

Diagram 97

Now place your fingers against your left wrist, as shown in Diagram 98. Notice that the third and fourth fingers are curled downward and hidden beneath the left wrist.

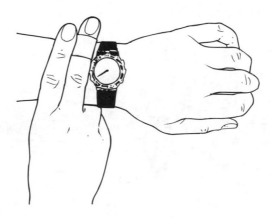

Diagram 98

Swing your hand upward about eighteen inches above the left wrist, as shown in Diagram 99.

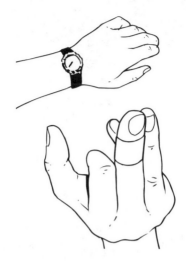

Diagram 99

As you bring your hand back down, change the positioning of your right fingers such that the second and third fingers become extended and the first and fourth fingers become curled. Immediately bring the hand down to the wrist again.

Your hands should look like the ones shown in Diagram 100.

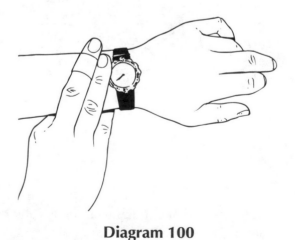

Diagram 100

Notice the right first and fourth fingers lodged under the wrist. Done at a quick pace, the illusion is that the band-aid transposed itself from one finger to another.

Finish by executing the move again, reversing your finger transposition to return to that shown in Diagram 98.

You can repeat this a couple times in rapid succession. Then simply show all your fingers, with the band-aid where it was all along—on the middle finger.

PROFESSIONAL TIP:

If you wear a watch on your left wrist, it adds another dimension to the communication of cognitive misinformation. This makes the illusion that much more difficult to figure out.

. . . .

"Every medical practice can use a little magic. It can lighten difficult days. Why not entertain while we try to comfort and cure?"

Robert Hogan, M.D.
Covina, CA

. . . .

CHAPTER 4

Items on Your Person

Using Your Fingers

Included here are a few effects that can be done without any type of prop. Nothing is needed but the fingers of your hands.

On Again, Off Again

✖ Rapport builder

⚀ Game

🗨 Clinical reasoning and thinking assessment

⧖ Time-saver

☺ Just for fun

① Skill level

PREFACE:

This is an oldie, but it still tickles the mind of the very young.

FX:

When the patient's mom explains how, while playing in the backyard, her son got his finger caught in the folding chair—imagine this scenario:

"Oh, that happened to me when I was your age. The doctor fixed it for me, and to this day, my finger works like magic. Wanna see?"

Continue by seemingly removing your finger from your hand, and then immediately replacing it.

EXPLANATION:

Proceed with the following demonstration. Then, when you complete your exhibition, ask the patient if you can look at *his or her* finger.

Finger Removal and Replacement:

1) Hold your right hand straight out and bend the index finger at the first joint, to about a 90° angle.

2) Now wrap the right middle and index fingers around the thumb. Your hand should resemble the one shown in Diagram 101.

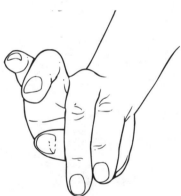

Diagram 101

3) By simply moving the left hand into the position shown in Diagram 102, you are set to begin. Simply move the right hand forward and then back. It creates the impression that the left index finger is being taken off and replaced. See Diagrams 102 and 103.

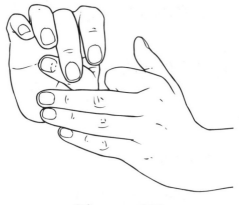

Diagram 102

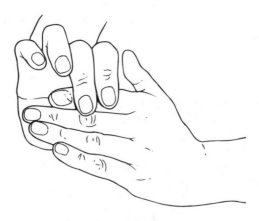

Diagram 103

PROFESSIONAL TIP:

More than once we've been told that the *Missing Finger* and the following finger stunts are ideal illusions for paramedics and EMTs! Next time you respond to a call with your hands full of first response equipment, rest easy. The necessary magical apparatus is always right there at hand...literally!

Paralyzed Finger

✖   Rapport builder

⚄   Game

🦗   Clinical reasoning and thinking assessment

🕷   Clinical motor skill experiment

⌛   Time-saver

①   Skill level

PREFACE:

With this one, the child does all the work. It is an excellent rapport builder, and enables you to play a little game to relax the patient before your exam.

Fx:

Once the patient's hands are placed according to your instructions, he or she will be unable to move the finger you select.

EXPLANATION:

First, ask the patient to cross his or her wrists. Then have the child interweave his or her fingers as shown in Diagram 104.

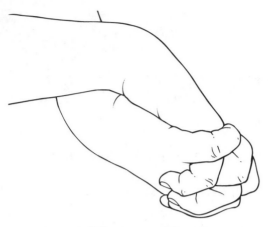

Diagram 104

Once in this position, have the child raise his or her hands so they are pointed upward, resembling the illustration in Diagram 105.

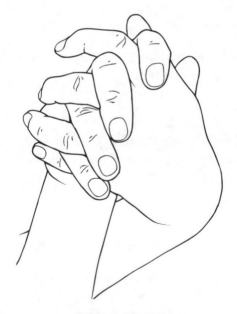

Diagram 105

As you point to one of his or her fingers, and ask the child to move it, he or she won't be able to do it.

PROFESSIONAL TIP:

This is a terrific experiment to demonstrate the left cerebral hemisphere's control of the right side of the body. Some doctors use this experiment to explain to family members the frustration that accompanies temporary paralysis in a stroke victim.

. . . .

"The idea of creating joy, laughter, play, and the ease with which these tools are readily accessible to the medical practitioner is long overdue. I celebrate the creativity of these little but effective tips for connection and silliness. This manual should become a classic."

Janet Thatcher Adams, M.D.
Clinical Professor, Department of
Family Practice and Community Health
University of Minnesota Medical School
Minneapolis, MN

. . . .

Finger Math

✖ Rapport builder

🎲 Game

🧠 Clinical reasoning and thinking assessment

⧗ Time-saver

① Skill level

PREFACE:

Here is another game that is designed to relax the child by getting his mind off the exam. It is fun and quick; ideal for those jam-packed days. As an alternative to the previous effect, try this. Here we assume that the patient not only is able to count to ten but also knows how to do simple addition and subtraction.

Fx:

Explain that most everyone knows that ten minus two equals eight. But not too many know that sometimes ten minus two can equal seven.

EXPLANATION:

Dovetail your hands such that the middle finger of the right hand is resting on the palm of the left hand, as shown in Diagram 106.

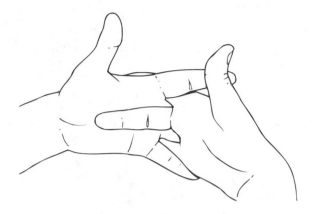

Diagram 106

The patient's view will be as shown in Diagram 107.

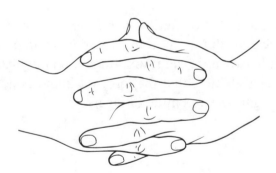

Diagram 107

Tell the patient that you just found out that ten minus two equals seven, which the patient will surely doubt if he or she knows their math. Say, *"Look. I have ten fingers, don't I? If I lower my thumbs* (lower your thumbs behind your hands, to hide them from the child's view), *that's ten minus two, right?"*

When the patient concurs that ten fingers minus two thumbs is the same as ten minus two, ask. *"How many fingers does that leave?"*

Clearly, the response will be, "Eight."

Say, *"Remember when I said that ten minus two can sometimes equal seven? I only have seven fingers. Count them for yourself."*

Because of the finger hidden in the palm, the patient will only be able to count seven, proving your modern math to be correct.

PROFESSIONAL TIP:

This is similar to the earlier trick, *It Floats* (page 101), in that you will have to adjust your mind's inclination to place the left first finger between the right first finger and thumb. Study the diagram again. Notice that the left first finger is actually between the right first and middle fingers.

More Finger Math

✖   Rapport builder

🎲   Game

💬   Clinical reasoning and thinking assessment

⏳   Time-saver

①   Skill level

PREFACE:

In this scenario, instead of showing your patient that you have only seven fingers, you explain that *he* or *she* has eleven fingers. Bear in mind that this is for the patient who is old enough to count to ten.

Fx:

State that the youngster has eleven fingers. When he or she assures you that there are only ten, present your new *fancy math*.

Have the patient hold out both hands with fingers extended. This not only will be the beginning of your magic counting procedure, but it will also allow you to get a cursory look at the patient's wounded finger.

Starting with the child's left hand, begin counting backwards. *"Ten, Nine, Eight, Seven, Six...."* As you count, touch each finger with your own finger. After saying *"Six,"* move your attention to the child's other hand, saying, *"And five makes eleven."*

This provides a perfect segue for you to apparently notice the patient's injured finger and complete your exam.

PROFESSIONAL TIP:

While this in no way is an official part of a typical psychological exam, it sure is a wonderful technique to nonchalantly ascertain a patient's cognitive and communication skills. It also presents a window to a patient's clinical reasoning and aptitude.

After demonstrating this stunt, it's best to just sit there quietly and not say anything. The uncomfortable sense of silence will force your patient to utter the first word. Typically, the patient will think for a moment and then ask you, "How did you do that?" The best retort is to ask the patient to explain how *he* or *she* thinks you did it.

. . . .

"These techniques will increase feelings of connection and rapport between caregiver and patient and serve to improve communication and enhance the quality of service."

Patty Wooten, R.N.
Santa Cruz, CA

. . . .

Still More Finger Math

✗   Rapport builder

▣   Game

◀   Clinical reasoning and thinking assessment

⧗   Time-saver

①   Skill level

PREFACE:

Our good friend Dr. Elliot Weinstein, of Montclair, California, used this method to teach children how to multiply by 9. It is highly interactive, allows the child to participate by calling out a number, and teaches the child a little math trick.

When learning the multiplication tables, kids find it very easy to learn the 10s, but they have greater difficulty learning the 9s. In this piece we take what is easy for them and use it to teach them what is more difficult for them.

Fx:

The attending nurse or physician uses his or her fingers to demonstrate how to multiply a given number, from 1 to 10, by 9.

EXPLANATION:

Using both hands, hold out your 10 fingers, as shown in Diagram 108.

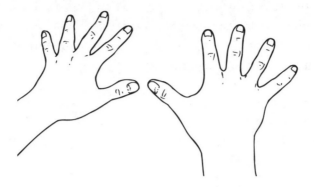

Diagram 108

The basic formula is simple. Beginning with the pinky finger
of the right hand, you will count from the right to the left. Count
off a finger for each number you tally. When you reach the
number stated by the patient, bend that finger downward. Let's
assume the child calls out the number 3. Starting with the little
finger and counting it as 1, the ring finger will be 2, and the
middle finger will be 3. Now simply bend the middle finger
down, as shown in Diagram 109.

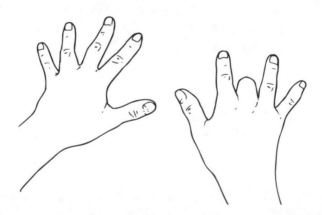

Diagram 109

Notice the two fingers to the right of the bent middle finger. Any fingers to the right of the bent finger (in this case two fingers) will count as 10 each. Any fingers to the left of the bent finger are simply added, counting each as 1.

We have 2 extended fingers to the right of the bent middle finger, so that gives us 20 (10 x 2 = 20). We have 7 extended fingers to the left of the bent middle finger, so that gives us 7. Now we simply add: 20 + 7 = 27. It's quite easy and very fast.

Let's try another number. Assume the child calls for the number 7. Counting from right to left, we run out of fingers on the right hand, so we continue our count onto the left. Ultimately, we end up having to bend the index finger of the left hand, as shown in Diagram 110.

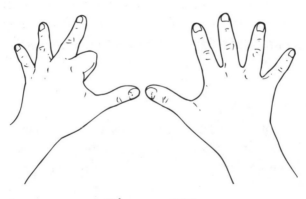

Diagram 110

You will notice that there are 6 extended fingers to the right of the bent left index finger: 10 x 6 = 60. There are 3 extended fingers to the left of the bent index finger, so we add: 3 + 60 = 63.

Frustrated Fingers

✖ Rapport builder

🎲 Game

🦴 Clinical motor skill experiment

① Skill level

PREVIEW:

This simple quickie is guaranteed to focus the patient away from the stress of the exam. It is a puzzle the patient will not be able to solve.

RESULTS:

The patient assistant to your demonstration finds it impossible to move his or her fingers.

EXPLANATION:

Have your patient make a pair of fists and place them together, face to face, palms down, knuckle to knuckle. Then both ring fingers should be extended upwards so that the fingertips touch.

It may take a little instruction to get the patient's hands positioned to duplicate that of the illustration shown in Diagram 111.

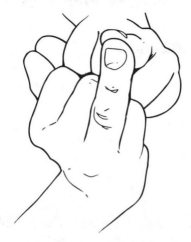

Diagram 111

However, once the patient's hands are properly set, you will be ready. Explain that the knuckles must continue touching. Now, no matter how hard the patient tries, he or she will not be able to move the fingers apart. It is a physical impossibility.

Professional Tip:

Be sure to use the ring fingers and the middle fingers. Some doctors teach the patient how to do this with the ring fingers. Then, as an added zinger, they perform the trick, substituting the middle fingers, which allows for success.

Eye Test

✖ Rapport builder

🗨 Clinical reasoning and thinking assessment

⧗ Time-saver

① Skill level

PREVIEW:

This effect requires no advance setup. It's a great time-saver, and your child patient will get a kick out of it. It can also prove to be an ideal time killer while the patient waits in the examining room.

Fx:

Upon executing your instructions, or those of your assistant, the patient sees the ends of his or her fingers combined to form a floating nub.

EXPLANATION:

This effect is a simple optical illusion.

Have the patient hold both hands out about three inches or so from his or her eyes. The index fingers should each point towards the other. Have the child bring the fingertips together until they touch.

Now comes the fun part. Tell the patient to look straight ahead, keeping both eyes opened, and to move the index fingers apart very slowly, as shown in Diagram 112. Instruct the patient to look past the fingers. By focusing beyond the obvious, the patient will be able to see the result.

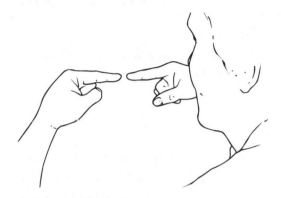

Diagram 112

The child may start to giggle, because he or she will begin to see a small, floating sausage-like substance floating between the fingers.

Again, this is more of a scientific fact than a bit of chicanery. What happens is this: It's not that our eyes and associated neurons are seeing anything unusual. In fact, to the eyes, there's nothing mysterious about an optical image. The deception arises when the image is processed by the brain. It is in the brain's interpretation that an image appears to be something else. Often this is based on the brain's merging of both the left and right images from the eyes into one image. This merging allows many ways to fool the brain into thinking it is seeing something that, in fact, it is not.

An example would be 3-D glasses. There's nothing 3-D about the glasses until a red filter is used for one lens and a blue filter for the other. Then your brain tries to combine it into one image. It is this combination that makes the image appear to be three-dimensional.

In this effect, the right eye sees the right fingertip and the left eye sees the left fingertip. Because the patient is looking straight ahead, both fingertips will remain in his or her vision as the fingers move apart. The result is a floating nub. Try it on yourself.

. . . .

"When I first started using these effects, my staff was initially upset with me for taking the time from my busy office. Let me tell you that now when we have an apprehensive child my staff come running to me to perform a bit of magic. Once the child gains confidence in me it actually speeds up my operation, making it more efficient."

Frank Kardos, M.D., P.A.
Wayne, NJ

. . . .

Wiggly Fingers

✖ Rapport builder

⚅ Game

🗨 Clinical reasoning and thinking assessment

⧗ Time-saver

① Skill Level

PREVIEW:

Here is another great time-saver that you can do on the fly.

RESULT:

The child patient gets a perplexing view of your two middle fingers wiggling in a very uncharacteristic fashion.

EXPLANATION:

We'll break this down into an easy set of steps.

First, place your palms together and bend your two middle fingers so that they point in opposite directions. See Diagram 113.

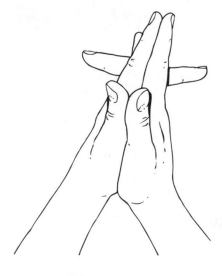

Diagram 113

Now rotate your palms, keeping all your other fingers straight. See Diagram 114.

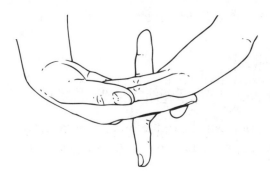

Diagram 114

You'll notice that only the middle fingers are interlocked. Now all that's left is to wiggle both middle fingers simultaneously.

Handkerchief Magic

Melting Knot

✗   Rapport builder

💬   Clinical reasoning and thinking assessment

①   Skill level

PREFACE:
Your pocket handkerchief or a scarf can provide an interesting interlude with the patient.

Fx:
A knot seems to melt off the handkerchief.

EXPLANATION:
Follow the illustrations below with a handkerchief in hand and just do everything as you read. It's quite easy.

Start by holding one end of the hanky between the first and second fingers of the left hand. See Diagram 115.

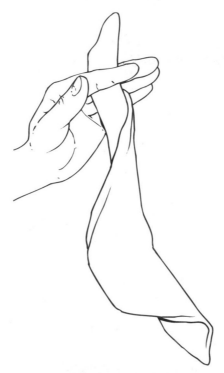

Diagram 115

With your right hand, bring the bottom end up, running it behind the hand, then between and through your left second and
third fingers. Continue through the crotch of the thumb, squeez-
ing the hanky between the thumb and first finger of the left
hand. Done correctly, your position will be like that illustrated
in Diagram 116.

Make sure that your left hand keeps a tight grip with its second
and third fingers. In the diagram, we have left a separation of these
fingers for clarity. But in practice they pinch against each other.

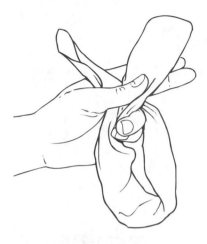

Diagram 116

Your right hand reaches through the loop that hangs beneath the left hand, and the fingers grab the end—marked X in Diagram 117.

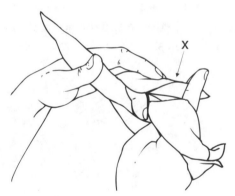

Diagram 117

The right fingers now pull this end through the loop and toward you. Keep a tight grip on the hanky in two spots. Spot 1 is the area between the left middle and ring fingers. Spot 2 is the area between the left thumb and first finger. See Diagram 118.

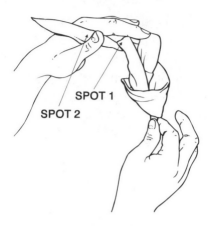

Diagram 118

Continue pulling on the end held by your right fingers. As the knot tightens, let it free up from the left-hand middle and ring fingers but not from the thumb and index finger. You can pull the ends to create the illusion of the knot. But don't pull too far or too fast because the knot will become undone. Rather, pull the ends just enough so the semblance of a knot appears in the middle of the hanky, as shown in Diagram 119.

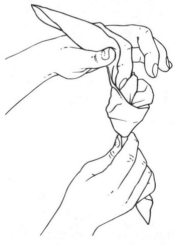

Diagram 119

All that is left is to ask your patient if he or she can count to three. When the proud announcement is that counting to three is easy, show your melting knot. As the counting proceeds, pull both ends away from the center, and the knot will dissolve, leaving you in the position illustrated in Diagram 120.

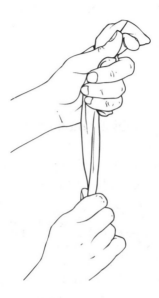

Diagram 120

PROFESSIONAL TIP:

You may want to explain to the child with a cough or cold the value of using a handkerchief. After all, when you had the sniffles and used your hanky, it suddenly became magical. Don't underestimate the value of having the child interact in the counting process. It is very powerful, and aligns you and the child patient. And THAT will make your job of treating the patient a whole lot easier.

The whole process of tying the knot and dissolving it should take no more than a few seconds.

Coin through Handkerchief

✖ Rapport builder

🗨 Clinical reasoning and thinking assessment

① Skill level

PREFACE:
In addition to a handkerchief, you'll need a quarter. This is fairly easy to perform, and can be done quickly, once mastered.

FX:
A coin seems to penetrate right through the cloth of the handkerchief. Upon examination, there is neither a hole in the hanky, nor anything unusual about the coin.

EXPLANATION:
Make sure the patient is seated to your left side. Hold a quarter in your left fingertips. Cover it with your hanky, making sure your hanky is not so transparent that the coin can be seen through it. You will need to execute a secret move here. When you drape the coin with the hanky, secure a bit of cloth between your thumb and the bottom of the coin. See Diagram 121. Notice there is a little extra cloth beneath the coin and the thumb.

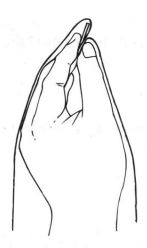

Diagram 121

But you will need to do another secret move. You want to show the patient that the coin is still there. So lift the side of the hanky that is nearest to the child. See Diagram 122.

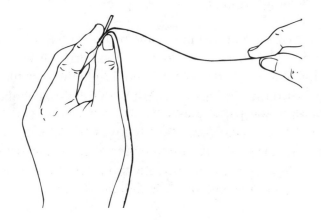

Diagram 122

Here's the last secret move. After showing that the coin is still in your fingertips, toss your hand forward and downward. You will want both the front AND the back of the hanky to fall over your hand. It will look perfectly fair, but the coin will now be outside the hanky, as shown in Diagram 123. All you have to do is make sure that you keep the hanky side toward the patient.

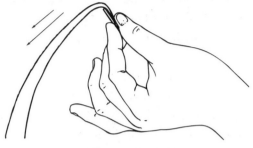

Diagram 123

Continue by twisting all the cloth that is below the coin. The contour of the coin will be apparent through the cloth. You can even slam it against the examining table to prove the coin is inside the hanky.

Give the twisted bottom ends to the patient and ask him or her to hold tightly. When the child has a good grip, slowly use the fingertips of both hands to rub the coin right through the handkerchief, as shown in Diagram 124. We've eliminated the view of the child's hands for clarity.

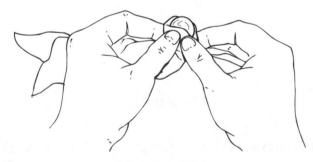

Diagram 124

Once the coin has penetrated the cloth, you can open the hanky to show that there are no holes or trap doors.

PROFESSIONAL TIP:

For being such a good assistant, give the quarter to the child, saying, "This *is a magic quarter, and if you put it under your pillow tonight, it will turn into a dollar.*"

Turn to the patient's parent or guardian and give them a wink and a nod to confirm that they have a job to do tonight. You may want to privately reinforce to the parent (verbally or with a note) the importance of complying with your little game.

All this sounds like fun, and it is. However, the bigger picture is that you will have a happy patient who will be excited about the next trip to the doctor.

Dentists may want to try this effect with a plastic-coated bib instead of a handkerchief.

. . . .

Here's one good doctor who agrees with us:

"Kids love to see things disappear. Giving the child the coin as a souvenir is a must."

Walter A. Schroeder, Jr., D.O, M.D., F.A.C.S.
Cape Girardeau, MO

. . . .

Coin Magic

All you'll need for the effects in this section is a small coin like a quarter. By reaching into your pocket, you'll be reaching for a tool that will intrigue the child patient, paving the way to your exam.

Vanishing Coin

✗   Rapport builder

⊕   Examination aid

🗨   Clinical reasoning and thinking experiment

☑   You've just done the exam

⧗   Time-saver

②   Skill level

PREVIEW:

You'll have to spend a little time learning what magicians call *The French Drop*. It is one of the easiest and most basic sleight-of-hand moves. It's ideal for the effect shown here.

Fx:

As the title indicates, a coin seems to disappear from your hand.

EXPLANATION:

The disappearance is not limited to coins (any small object will do). But for the purposes of discussion, let's stay with a coin.

Begin by holding the coin by its edges between the thumb and middle finger of the right hand. The left hand now reaches for the coin with the thumb being inserted into the left hand, and beneath the coin. See Diagram 125.

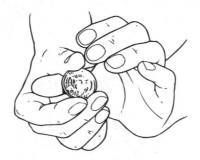

Diagram 125

Pretend to grab the coin with the right hand, but secretly allow it to fall into the left palm, as exposed in Diagram 126.

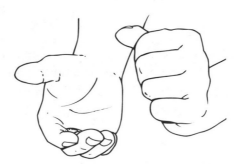

Diagram 126

In practice, you will curl the right-hand fingers a bit upward. Simultaneously, while keeping the left hand tightly closed, address your attention to it as if it holds the coin. This is accomplished by continuing to curl your right hand and using it to point to the left, as shown in Diagram 127.

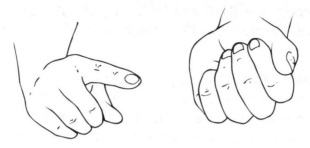

Diagram 127

Now slowly open the left hand, showing that the coin has vanished.

"Where could it be? Let me check your ear. It's not there. Maybe it's in the other ear. It's not there either. Maybe it's in your mouth. Open wide. Nope. It's not there." Guess what? You've just checked the child's ears and mouth.

PROFESSIONAL TIP:

Just as with the otoscope that we talked about earlier, the coin provides an excellent technique to initiate an exam of the child's ears, nose, and throat. We recommend finding the coin by pulling it into view from the back of the child's head.

Physicians wash their hands frequently (hopefully). Coins are handled more easily when the palms are dry. A minimal amount of moisture can create enough surface tension for a coin to "stick," or hang up temporarily. This could make the *French Drop* move appear cumbersome. Dry hands are better for handling coins. However, you don't want them to be too dry. Experiment to find what works best for you.

Coin Appearance

We're sure you will come up with many ways to reproduce the coin from the previous effect. But here are a few suggestions:

1) Grab a cotton ball and place it over the coin. Now push the coin up through the cotton. (If you have to give the child an injection, this would be a nice prelude to reaching for another cotton ball to swab his or her arm).

2) Tug on the patient's earlobe. Then slide the coin to your fingertips before you bring it into view. (An excellent way to begin an ear exam).

3) With the coin concealed in your hand, turn the hand palm down. Gently squeeze the child's nose with your thumb and index finger. Allow the coin to drop and catch it with your other hand. Then say, *"Let me take a look to see what else you have up that nose!*

Coin from Elbow

This is ideal for the patient who comes in with a bad wing. As you enter the examining room, or at a point when the patient is looking somewhere other than at you, secretly place a quarter in the crotch of your left elbow. Keep your arm slightly bent so the coin does not dislodge.

While maintaining the arms in a bent posture, explain that after you injured your own arm when you were the patient's age, it became a money machine, and every day your elbow produces a quarter.

Show both hands empty. Now rub your left elbow with your right hand. Secretly grasp the coin into the right hand, keeping it hidden. It is best to use the right thumb to slide the coin into the right palm from the crotch formed by the bent arm. Continue rubbing the elbow. A moment later, open your hand and show the coin.

If you do this in a mirror a couple of times, you'll have it down in no time.

Flying Penny

✖ Rapport builder

☑ You've just done the exam

⚍ Time-saver

① Skill level

PREVIEW:

Now that you have learned the *French Drop*, here's an easy, fun item. You will need two things: *two* pennies (similar in appearance) and an empty matchbox. This effect is so good that if you don't have a matchbox, you may want to go out and get one.

RESULT:

A penny disappears in your elbow and reappears inside a matchbox, which was previously shown as empty.

EXPLANATION:

There is a little advance setup to this piece. Begin by wedging one of the pennies between the back edge of the matchbox drawer and the top of the box. It should be just out of sight and held into place by the matchbox itself. To the casual eye, the matchbox will appear to be empty. Show the spectator your matchbox and mention that it is nothing more than an empty matchbox, which you will get back to later. Explain, *"It is empty because matches are very dangerous and can make a fire. And nobody should ever play with matches."* You can show the box in a casual manner, as shown in Diagram 128.

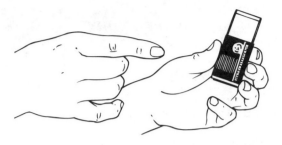

Diagram 128

When showing the matchbox, be gentle. If you are, you can turn the box upside down and sideways without fear of dislodging the coin. Then set the box on the examining table, away from the patient. It should look like the illustration shown in Diagram 129.

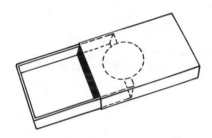

Diagram 129

Now close the box with one hand on each end. This will cause the penny to fall inside the drawer-like box. Once this is completed, you are all set to mystify the child.

Reach into your pocket and remove the matching penny. Explain that it is actually a magical penny. Now you must execute the *French Drop* that you learned earlier. Hold the penny in the left hand and pretend to take it with the right. The penny actually falls into the waiting left fingers. Without pause, lift your left arm and bring your right hand to the left elbow.

Say, *"If I rub the coin into my elbow it will disappear."*

Remove your right fingers and show your right hand empty. Check your elbow for the coin. Now put both hands into your lab coat pockets, as if to see if the penny is there. This is a ploy to enable you to leave the penny that is in the left hand in the left pocket.

Bring out your hands totally empty. Here you can go into an examination of the child's ears, nose, and throat (similar to what was described in *The Vanishing Coin*). Once your exam is finished and you've exhausted all possible locations for the missing penny, continue as follows. *"Wait! Remember the little box?"* Reach over and pick up the box with one hand. Shake it. The coin will dislodge and lay in the box, as shown in Diagram 130. Continue shaking the box so the child can hear the coin rattle inside. Hand the box to the patient to open.

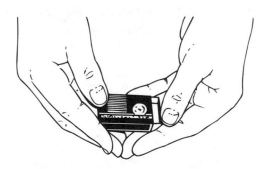

Diagram 130

Let the patient keep the penny if his or her age is appropriate. As we mentioned earlier, you don't want a toddler to have any small object that could be swallowed.

PROFESSIONAL TIP:

This is another excellent way to complete an exam under what the child sees as fun circumstances. Additionally, you are educating the patient about not playing with matches. The child will be having so much fun as you search for the penny that he or she will not even be aware that the examination is taking place.

This is an excellent trick for medically trained firefighters and paramedics. One firefighter we know uses this to open his speech on fire safety to fifth graders.

· ·

"...Health-care providers can become the STAR, mastering some of the 'right moves' that magically and dramatically set the stage to 'get in touch' with their own audience/patients. With the right effect, an office visit can actually become fun, funny and entertaining! Curtain Up! You're ON!"

Dale Anderson, M.D., F.A.C.S., D.A.B.H.M.
St. Paul, MN

· ·

Easy Come, Easy Go

✖ Rapport builder

⌛ Time-saver

① Skill level

PREFACE:

This effect requires some advance preparation: You need a quarter, and two pennies that are similar in appearance.

Take a small piece of scotch tape and place it on one of the pennies, being careful that the tape does not overlap the coin. Now stick the penny to the quarter. See Diagram 131.

Diagram 131

Keep the quarter (with attached penny) and the loose penny in your pocket until you are ready to perform.

Fx:

This is another disappearance of a coin. The advantage here is that you will be left with an empty hand.

EXPLANATION:

When ready, remove the coins from your pocket, being careful not to expose the hidden penny. Place the quarter in the palm of your left hand so that the penny remains hidden beneath it. Then place the loose penny atop the quarter, as shown in Diagram 132.

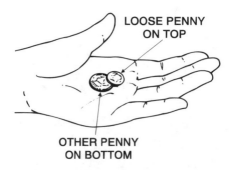

LOOSE PENNY
ON TOP

OTHER PENNY
ON BOTTOM

Diagram 132

Show your coins to the spectator, saying, *"I have a penny and a quarter, right?"* When the eagle-eyed patient agrees, openly remove the loose penny with the right hand and place it into your right pocket.

"And if I put a penny in my pocket, what do I have left?" Confidently, the child will reply, "A quarter."

In the process of opening your left hand, flip the (double) coin so the penny side is up. The youngster will see a quarter and a penny. You will say, *"No. I have a quarter and a penny."*

Now again close your hand around the coin(s). Allow enough room for your right hand to reach in and pull out the taped quarter. Be sure to openly remove the quarter, remembering to keep the left hand closed so that the taped penny is behind it and out of the patient's view. Place it in your right pocket with the previously deposited penny. *"If I remove the quarter, what do I have left?"*

The patient will respond, "A penny." Open your left hand and show it empty. Say, *"Easy come, easy go."*

PROFESSIONAL TIP:

Several physicians we've talked to say they use this following surgery or on hospital rounds. *"The anesthesia may change how you see money."* Follow through with the trick. Then explain that you'll check again tomorrow.

The next day, repeat the trick but let the patient "win" by removing the tape during the last move.

For a more permanent magic coin, try a spot of super glue or permanent bonding material in place of the tape.

CHAPTER 5

Items in Your Office

Miscellaneous Office Magic

Y our office has an array of items that can be used to capture the interest of the child patient. We've selected a few of our favorites.

Hole in the Hand Illusion

✖ Rapport builder

🗨 Clinical reasoning and thinking assessment

☺ Just for fun

① Skill level

PREVIEW:

This is nice and quick. The preparation is easy. Once completed, you will be set for many, many performances. Simply take a piece of 8 1/2 x 11-inch binder paper, roll it into a tube, and tape it securely. The diameter of the tube should be about one inch. This effect also provides an introduction to examining the patient more thoroughly.

RESULT:

Looking through a paper tube, the patient sees a hole in his or her hand.

EXPLANATION:

This is an optical illusion. Hand the tube to your patient, instructing that it be held up to his or her right eye. Keeping both eyes open, the child should bring his or her left hand up alongside the tube. The patient will see a hole in his or her left hand. This is illustrated in Diagram 133.

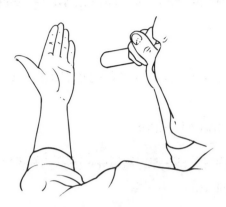

Diagram 133

This works, not because of any ruse—it is basic science. When a person looks at something, each eye sees the item separately. The brain brings the two images together to form a single image. Because of the tube and the close proximity of the hand, the brain is unable to form a single image of the hand. Thus, the hole appears.

PROFESSIONAL TIP:

For a prefashioned tube, look no further than the empty tube from a roll of paper towels.

Radiological technicians have told us that this illusion helps serve as a way to explain the differences in diagnostic modalities available today.

No More Elephants

✖ Rapport builder

☻ Just for fun

① Skill level

PREVIEW:

This is just pure fun. It is more what comedians and magicians call *a bit* than an actual trick.

EXPLANATION:

If you have table paper, you are left with the long rolls when the paper has all been used. Take a roll, pucker your lips tightly (inside either end), and blow. With practice, this can produce a sound remarkably like an elephant. Kids love the sound and try to duplicate your efforts, usually without success. Explain to the patient, *"This scares away elephants."* When the patient laughs or questions your reasoning, ask, *"Have you seen even one in my office?"*

Jumping Rubber Band

✗   Rapport builder

🗨   Clinical reasoning and thinking assessment

🐾   Clinical motor skill experiment

⧗   Time-saver

①   Skill level

ABOUT PROJECT MAGIC AND THERAPY

Project Magic began in 1982, when magician David Copperfield realized that patients undergoing physical rehabilitation could benefit greatly by mixing magical sleight-of-hand tricks with today's medicine.

After a debilitating stroke or a car accident, a patient's recovery is often dependent on weeks or months of physical and occupational therapy. Many times this rehabilitation is an exhausting process that can seem unrewarding and downright difficult for the patient. For some, the goal is to simply tie a shoe, zip a zipper, or take a step or two—but imagine if these same patients could increase their real-world dexterity while learning a nimble-fingered magic trick instead. The patients would finish their therapy session with the motivation to practice their skills on their own time and show off their new magical abilities to friends and family. Patients would finish their rehabilitation with the ability to do something special and unique. They could perform magic tricks that no one else could do. Imagine the psychological benefits to this approach, as well as the increased self-esteem…and the rewards would obviously go far beyond the physical!

This magical approach to therapy works equally well for older adults who want to learn an effect or two to show their grandchildren, and for younger patients who can't wait to show off their newly mastered skill to a fellow patient, a parent, or a friend. From a stroke victim who needs to work on fine motor skills to a quadriplegic who masters a mind-reading effect, magic and therapy can—and do—go hand in hand.

Project Magic isn't limited to physical rehabilitation. Speech and occupational therapists use the performance of magic to increase cognitive function, enhance speech, improve self-esteem, reduce depression, and develop social skills.

The following effect, *The Jumping Rubber Band*, is a well-known trick to magicians, but it has seen new light in the hands of the therapists and patients involved in Project Magic. This effect is a perfect one for those who want to increase the fine motor skills involved in the opening and closing of a hand. As a health-care provider you may want to keep the secret of the jumping rubber band trick to yourself. However, if you would like to share the method in the scope of physical therapy, you may want to contact Project Magic directly to find out more about their unique program.

Project Magic is a not-for-profit organization that is governed by a board of directors, with internationally known illusionist David Copperfield as its active chairperson.

For more information please contact:

Project Magic
c/o Stormont-Vail West
3707 S.W. 6th Avenue
Topeka, KS 66606

PREVIEW:

This is a great time-saver, and it may be one that you'll want to teach the child patient to perform. All you need is a rubber band in the pocket of your lab coat, and you're set to begin.

FX:

A rubber band jumps from your first two fingers to your second two fingers.

EXPLANATION:

If you can secure a thick rubber band, even better. Hold your left hand upward with the palm facing you. Place the rubber band over your index and middle fingers at the knuckle, just below the second phalanx, as shown in Diagram 134.

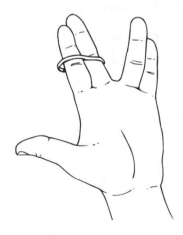

Diagram 134

Show both sides of your hand to the patient. Now allow the rubber band to slide down to the base of your fingers, just above the palm.

With your right hand, grasp the rubber band near the middle finger and stretch the band across the palm of your hand. Simultaneously, curl your left fingers downward and into the newly formed gap created by the stretched rubber band. See illustration in Diagram 135.

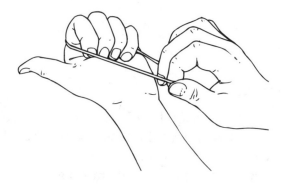

Diagram 135

Keep pulling the rubber band until it passes the baby finger of the left hand. Now let it fall over all four fingers. It must rest along the first phalanx near the base of your fingernails, as shown in Diagram 136.

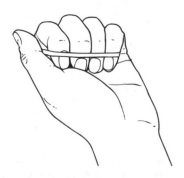

Diagram 136

Maintain a fist-like position with your hand, and turn it over with the knuckles upward. Here the rubber band appears to be wrapped around only your first two fingers. See Diagram 137.

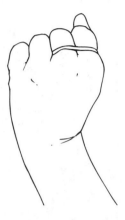

Diagram 137

You are now set for the magic jump. When you quickly straighten your fingers, the rubber band will automatically leap to the other two fingers, as shown in Diagram 138.

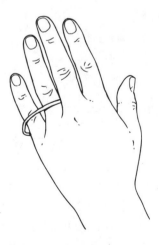

Diagram 138

PROFESSIONAL TIP:

Naturally, people should not know how the rubber band is placed in advance. With a minimal amount of practice, you will be able to set it up before revealing the enigma.

We've found that a rubber band that is between one and two inches long works best. You may want to teach this to your preteen patients. Having something special to show to their friends will expand their self-confidence.

. . . .

"...Great creativity is brought into the clinical exam room with an offering of several 'magic' pearls. I now routinely use a number of them and am eager for more."

Benjamin Cable, M.D.
Chief Pediatric Otolaryngology
Triplu Army Medical Hospital
Honolulu, HI

. . . .

Neck Penetration

✖ Rapport builder

⧗ Time-saver

① Skill level

PREVIEW:

Is the hand quicker than the eye? In this case it is.

Fx:

A length of twine seems to pass right through your neck.

EXPLANATION:

Take a length of string, approximately three- to four-feet long, and tightly tie off the ends to form a loop. Now place the loop around the back of your neck, holding each end with the first finger of each hand. See Diagram 139.

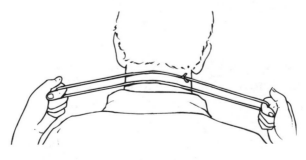

Diagram 139

Bring your hands together at the front of your neck to the point where the two ends are almost touching one another.

Now you must turn your hands to hide both the ends of the loop and your fingers, by placing the back of your hands toward the spectator. See Diagram 140.

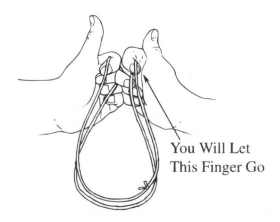

You Will Let
This Finger Go

Diagram 140

Tell the patient that you can cause the string to pass right through your neck. As you speak, slip your right-hand middle finger into the loop that is held by the left-hand index finger. You are now ready for the climax.

Allow your right index finger to come to the edge of the string so that it is hardly holding it. This puts you in a position to let go of the string quickly and effortlessly. Again, refer to Diagram 139.

Say to the patient, *"Ready? Now!"* Spread your hands wide apart, and the string will seem to have penetrated through your neck.

Diagram 141 shows the slight change in position. As you can see, the string is now on the right middle finger rather than the index finger, as when you started.

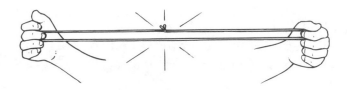

Diagram 141

Professional Tip:

This could also be done through your leg. The choice is yours. The method is the same. But if you think that very young patients are *too* young and could accidentally choke themselves, your leg may be a better choice.

Linking Paper Clips

✖ Rapport builder

🐦 Clinical reasoning and thinking assessment

① Skill level

PREVIEW:

All you'll need for this experiment are two paper clips and a sheet of paper from your prescription pad.

FX:

Two paper clips link themselves in what seems an impossible manner.

EXPLANATION:

Attach the paper clips to the folded paper as illustrated in Diagram 142, and they will link.

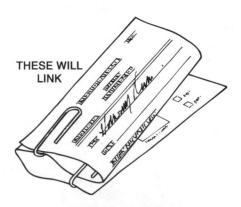

THESE WILL
LINK

Diagram 142

Note: If you attach the paper clips as shown in Diagram 143, they will not link. Study the difference between the two setups.

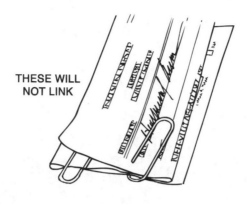

THESE WILL
NOT LINK

Diagram 143

Study the difference in how the two pieces of paper in Diagrams 142 and 143 are clipped. Try it both ways for yourself. Practice the setup a few times to get a feel for how to put the clips onto the paper. After a few attempts, you'll be doing it without a second thought.

Here's the performance.

Show the child patient a sheet from your prescription pad, along with two paper clips. Fold the paper and attach the paper clips as shown in Diagram 142. Once completed, grasp the paper by the ends as shown in Diagram 144.

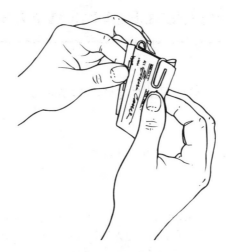

Diagram 144

All that's left is for you to tug outward on the two ends. As the paper stretches, the paper clips will automatically link and pop from the paper, as shown in Diagram 145.

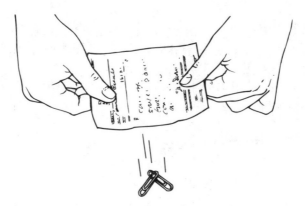

Diagram 145

The reason for explaining the attachment methods for both success and failure is this: In the event your patient wants to try it, you have the discretion relative to which outcome you would prefer, given the situation.

Side-Fx

PUZZLE ANSWERS

1) "Too wise you are, too wise you be, I see you are too wise for me."

2) As shown in Diagram 146, add a single line to make some of the "o's" into "g," "d," and "a." "good dog do a trick"

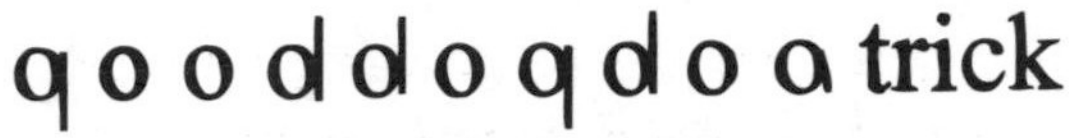

$$q\,o\,o\,d\,d\,o\,q\,d\,o\,a\,trick$$

Diagram 146

3) If you are to solve this puzzle, you must think outside the box. Imagine that there are two extra dots; this allows you to draw a triangle and one extra line. Examine Diagram 147.

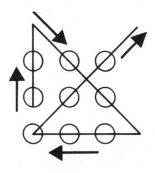

Diagram 147

4) Lemonade (Lem *on* ade)

5) Inside Information

6) 7-up can

7) I under STAND

Swab Swami Answers

Here are the answers for the puzzle questions on page 105.

1) From Diagram 72, add five swabs to spell "NINE." The answer is below in Diagram 148.

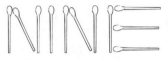

Diagram 148

2) Make them into Roman numerals: III (three) and VI (six, or one half dozen). See Diagram 149.

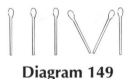

Diagram 149

3) From Diagram 73, using four swabs, make them spell "TEN." Refer to Diagram 150 for the solution.

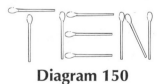

Diagram 150

4) From Diagram 74, make the swabs spell "NIL." See Diagram 151.

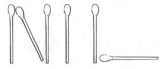

Diagram 151

5) Place the two triangles face to face as seen below in Diagram 152.

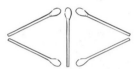

Diagram 152

6) Arrange the swabs as seen below in Diagram 153. If you only find four triangles, keep looking. There are five.

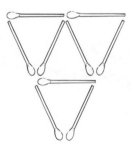

Diagram 153

SPECIAL THANKS

To Nancy, Linda, Lucas, and Stephanie for putting up with our sometimes obsessive quest to make this project a reality.

For all your help in changing a caterpillar into a butterfly:

Illustrations: Tony Dunn

Initial Photographs: Victor Trabucco

Graphics: Stan Holden

Icon Font Creations: James Grieshaber

Cover Photography: Greg Porter

Publishing: Susan A. Friedmann

Consulting: Chris Smith and Bucky Rosenbaum

Editing & Proofing: Norma J. Collins

Typesetting: Jim Weems and Barbara Weems

This book would not be possible without the enthusiasm and support of so many physicians from around the country. We would particularly like to extend our gratitude to:

Patch Adams, M.D., for his gusto and zeal in treating the human spirit as well as the human body…and for his motivation and inspiration to dream.

For your contributions, recommendations, comments, and investment of time:

Gary Grayman, M.D., M.B.A., C.P.E. F.A.C.E.P., Palm Springs, CA

Ralph Argen, M.D., F.A.C.P., Williamsville, NY

Robert Hogan, M.D., Covina, CA

Ellen Rabun, M.D., Blacksburg, VA

Elliot Weinstein, M.D., F.A.A.P., Montclair, CA

Walter Schroeder, D.O., M.D., F.A.C.S., Cape Girardeau, MO

Hector Ramirez, M.D., Rancho Santa Margarita, CA

Patricia Wopperer, R.N., M.S., C.N.O.R., East Amherst, NY

Robert Pyke, R.N., C.P.N.P., Cuyahoga Falls, OH

Alicia Bednar, R.N., West Hills, CA

Shobhana Schwebke, The Hospital Clown Newsletter. Oakland, CA

Leticia Garcia, Jennifer Waggoner, Aarah Haase, Rancho Santa Margarita, CA

Patricia Nabozny, Colden, NY

Julie DeJean, Topeka, KS

Gilbert L. Furman, M.D., Covina, CA

Bradford L. Waiters, M.D., F.A.C.E.P., Royal Oak, MI

Mark Criswell, M.D., El Paso, TX

Benjamin Cable, M.D., Honolulu, HI

Frank Kardos, M.D., P.A., Wayne, NJ

Robert W. Block, M.D., Tulsa, OK

Dale Anderson, M.D., F.A.C.S., D.A.B.H.M., St. Paul, MN

Dennis Guest, D.O., F.A.C.O.E.P., F.A.C.E.P., Philadelphia, PA

Jan Thatcher Adams, M.D., Minneapolis, MN

Patty Wooten, R.N., Santa Cruz, CA

Additional Thanks and Acknowledgments to:

Magician: David Copperfield and Project Magic.

Magicians: Giovanni Livera, Danny Orleans, Lubor Fiedler, Doug Bennett, Steve Cohen, Bill Okal, Looy Simonoff, Gary Darwin.

BIBLIOGRAPHY—
REFERENCES AND SOURCES

Books

Abraham, R.M. *Easy to Do Entertainment and Diversions*. New York: Dover Publishing, 1961.

Abraham, R.M. *Diversions and Pastimes*. New York: Dover Publishing, 1964.

Adams, Hunter, and Maureen Mylander. *Gesundheit*, Rochester: Healing Arts Press, 1993.

Adams, Patch, M.D. *House Calls*. San Francisco: Robert D. Reed Publishers, 1998.

Baker, Susan-Keane. *Managing Patient Expectations, The Art of Finding and Keeping Loyal Patients*. San Francisco: Jossey-Bass, 1998.

Bokun, Branko. *Humour Therapy*. London: Vita Books, 1986.

Christopher, Milbourne. *Panorama of Magic*. New York: Dover Publishing, 1962.

Copperfield, David. *Tales of the Impossible*. New York: Harper Prism, 1995.

Cousins, Norman. *Head First, The Biology of Hope and the Healing Power of the Human Spirit.* New York: Penguin Books, 1989.

Cousins, Norman. *Anatomy of an Illness as Perceived by the Patient.* New York: Bantam Books, 1981.

Davidson, Greg. *The Everything Magic Book.* Holbrook: Adams Media Corporation, 2000.

Desmond, Joanne, and Lanny R. Copeland. *Communicating with Today's Patient. Essentials to Save Time, Decrease Risk, and Increase Patient Compliance.* San Francisco: Jossey-Bass, 2000.

Dolan, Edward Jr. *Let's Make Magic.* New York: Doubleday & Company, 1981.

Dunninger, Joseph. *Dunninger's Complete Encyclopedia of Magic.* London: The Hamlyn Group Limited, 1967.

Fisher, John. *Never Give a Sucker an Even Break.* New York: Panteon Books, 1976.

Gerteis, Margaret, Susan Edgman-Levitan, Jennifer Daley, and Thomas L. Delbanco. *Through the Patient's Eyes, Understanding and Promoting Patient-Centered Care.* San Francisco: Jossey-Bass, 1993.

Gordon James, M.D. *Manifesto for Healing.* Reading: Addison-Wesley, 1996.

Hay, Henry. *Amateur Magician's Handbook.* New York: The New American Library, Inc., 1965.

Herz, Bill. *Secrets of Astonishing the Executive.* New York: Avon Publishing, 1991.

Ho, Oliver. *Amazing Math Magic.* New York: Sterling Publishing, 2001.

Holden, Robert. *Laughter is the Best Medicine.* London: Thorsons, 1993.

Keller, Charles. *Tongue Twisters.* New York: Simon & Schuster, 1989.

Kettelkamp, Larry. *Magic Made Easy.* New York: William Morrow & Company, 1981.

Livera, Giovanni, and Ken Press. *The Amazing Dad.* New York: Berkley Publishing, 2001.

Olney, Ross, and Pat Olney. *Easy to Make Magic.* New York: Random House, 1979.

Pogue, David, and Mark Levy. *Magic for Dummies.* Foster City: IDG Books Worldwide, 1998.

Roop, Peter, and Connie Roop. *Stick Out Your Tongue.* Minneapolis: Lerner Publishing, 1986.

Schindler, George. *Presto, Magic for the Beginner.* New York: Reiss Publishing, 1977.

Schwartz, Alan. *Unriddling, A Collection of American Folklore.* New York: Sterling Publishing, 1983.

Shalit, Gene. *Laughing Matters.* New York: Doubleday & Company, 1987.

Sloane, Paul, and Des MacHale. *Lateral Thinking Puzzles*. New York: Sterling Publishing, 1950.

Spiro, Howard, Mary G. McCrea Curnen, Enid Peschel, and Deborah St. James. *Empathy and the Practice of Medicine, Beyond Pills and the Scalpel*. New Haven: Yale University Press.

Stoddard, Edward. *The First Book of Magic*. New York: Franklin Watts Publishing, 1953.

Verno, Michael. *Camp Good Days A to Z Joke Book*. Children's Oncology Publications, 1998.

Wood, Elizabeth, and Shawn McMaster. *50 Super Magic Tricks*. New York: RGA Publishing, 1997.

Zaslove, Marshall O., M.D. *The Successful Physician, A Productivity Handbook for Practitioners*. Gaithersburg: Aspen Publishers, 2003.

Articles

"Practical Ways to Improve Patient Satisfaction with Visit Length." George E. Kikano, M.D., David A. Gross, M.S., and Kurt C. Strange, M.D., PhD. American Academy of Family Physicians, Family Practice Management, September 1999.

"Relationships between Physician Practice Style, Patient Satisfaction, and Attributes of Primary Care." Susan A. Flocke, William L. Miller, and Benjamin F. Crabtree. *The Journal of Family Practice*, October 2002.

"Empathy, Warmth Can Be Potent Medicine." Suzanne Rostler. The Lancelot, 357:757-762, 2001.

"The Biological Basis of the Placebo Effect." E. Russo. The Scientist, 16[24]:30-1, December 9, 2002.

"The Needlestick Safety and Prevention Act." HR 5178. September, 2000.

"Through the Hank." Martin Gardiner's Manuscript. The Jinx, Winter Extra, December 1937.

"Cute Coin." E.S. Hoffman. The Phoenix, March 19, 1943.

We would love to hear from you!

Have you been inspired or motivated to add magic to your practice? Do you have a magical idea that you would like to share with your colleagues? Perhaps you have a comment, concern, or a question about Side-Fx? Why not share your experiences with us…and the world!

There is more Side-Fx on the Web at

http://www.SideFxMagic.com

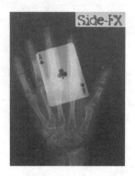

Email us at SideFx@CorporateFX.com

Or you can reach us by mail at:

**Side-FX
c/o Corporate-FX
P.O. Box 1624
Tustin, CA 92781-1624
United States of America**

By Telephone:

**Phone 1.714.731.4591
Toll-Free 1.800.MAGIC.13**

NOTES

NOTES

NOTES

NOTES